T0201867

Building Strategic Skills for Better Health

Building Strategic Skills for Better Health

A Primer for Public Health Professionals

Edited by
Michael R. Fraser, PhD, MS, CAE, FCPP
and
Brian C. Castrucci, DrPH, MA

de Beaumont
BOLD SOLUTIONS FOR HEALTHIER COMMUNITIES.

OXFORD
UNIVERSITY PRESS

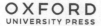

OXFORD
UNIVERSITY PRESS

Oxford University Press is a department of the University of Oxford. It furthers
the University's objective of excellence in research, scholarship, and education
by publishing worldwide. Oxford is a registered trade mark of Oxford University
Press in the UK and certain other countries.

Published in the United States of America by Oxford University Press
198 Madison Avenue, New York, NY 10016, United States of America.

© de Beaumont Foundation 2024

All rights reserved. No part of this publication may be reproduced, stored in
a retrieval system, or transmitted, in any form or by any means, without the
prior permission in writing of Oxford University Press, or as expressly permitted
by law, by license, or under terms agreed with the appropriate reproduction
rights organization. Inquiries concerning reproduction outside the scope of the
above should be sent to the Rights Department, Oxford University Press, at the
address above.

You must not circulate this work in any other form
and you must impose this same condition on any acquirer.

CIP data is on file at the Library of Congress

ISBN 978–0–19–774460–4

DOI: 10.1093/oso/9780197744604.001.0001

This material is not intended to be, and should not be considered, a substitute for medical or other
professional advice. Treatment for the conditions described in this material is highly dependent on
the individual circumstances. And, while this material is designed to offer accurate information with
respect to the subject matter covered and to be current as of the time it was written, research and
knowledge about medical and health issues is constantly evolving and dose schedules for medications
are being revised continually, with new side effects recognized and accounted for regularly. Readers
must therefore always check the product information and clinical procedures with the most up-to-date
published product information and data sheets provided by the manufacturers and the most recent codes
of conduct and safety regulation. The publisher and the authors make no representations or warranties
to readers, express or implied, as to the accuracy or completeness of this material. Without limiting the
foregoing, the publisher and the authors make no representations or warranties as to the accuracy or
efficacy of the drug dosages mentioned in the material. The authors and the publisher do not accept, and
expressly disclaim, any responsibility for any liability, loss, or risk that may be claimed or incurred as a
consequence of the use and/or application of any of the contents of this material.

Printed by Marquis Book Printing, Canada

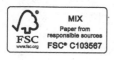

To the countless public servants, public health leaders, health professionals, and private-sector partners who work tirelessly to keep America healthy: We thank you for your service.

Contents

Acknowledgments

Developing a volume like this one is a collective endeavor, and we appreciate the work of the many contributors and staff who spent their valuable time and effort to make this book a useful tool for the public health workforce. In particular, we would like to acknowledge our authors, who donated their expertise and their precious time to prepare each chapter and worked collaboratively with us to finalize them. This book also would not have been possible without the editorial support, project management, and expertise of Dena Afrasiabi, Zamir M. Brown, Sarah Canty, Grace Castillo, Julia Haskins, Emma Hodgdon, Sarah Humphreville, J.T. Lane, Diane Lazarus, Nalini Padmanabhan, Greg Papillon, Joseph Parsons, Blair Reynolds, and Katie Sellers. We sincerely thank you for your counsel, partnership, and dedication to public health.

Contributors

Manal J. Aboelata, MPH, Deputy Executive Director of Prevention Institute

Manal J. Aboelata is the deputy executive director of Prevention Institute, a national nonprofit dedicated to advancing strategies to achieve health equity, prevent illness and injury, and ensure safe and healthy communities. An epidemiologist by training, Manal advocates for health equity and racial justice. She writes and speaks on many issues, especially those pertaining to health equity and the built environment. Manal co-authored a chapter in the first and second editions of *Making Healthy Places* and wrote the foreword to *Schools That Heal: Design with Mental Health in Mind*. She has written numerous original articles, op-eds, and policy briefs on timely, relevant public health justice issues. Manal has served on numerous health advisory boards, review panels, and expert councils.

Manal earned her master's degree in public health with a concentration in epidemiology from the University of California, Los Angeles, and her Bachelor of Arts degree from the University of California, Berkeley. Manal was inducted into the UCLA School of Public Health Hall of Fame in 2009 and was a Stanton Fellow of the Durfee Foundation from 2017 to 2019.

Mayela Arana, MPH, CHES, CPH, Associate Director of the Region 2 Public Health Training Center at the Columbia University Mailman School of Public Health

Mayela Arana is the associate director of the Region 2 Public Health Training Center at Columbia University's Mailman School of Public Health and the co-chair of the Public Health Training Center Network's Racial Justice Workgroup. Mayela works to ensure that the current and future public health workforce is adequately trained to address emerging health challenges, and her expertise lies at the intersection of public health practice and academic research. Prior to this work, Mayela worked for the New York City Health + Hospitals Partnerships for Early Childhood Development grant to address social determinants of health in pediatric settings, and the USDA-funded

Starting Early Obesity Prevention Program, specifically focused on nutrition education and food insecurity among Hispanic families.

Mayela holds a Master of Public Health with a concentration in health promotion, research, and practice from Columbia University's Mailman School of Public Health and a Bachelor of Arts in psychology from the University of San Francisco.

Kyle Bogaert, MPH, Senior Director for Performance Excellence at the Association of State and Territorial Health Officials

Kyle Bogaert is the senior director for performance excellence at the Association of State and Territorial Health Officials (ASTHO), the national nonprofit membership association representing the leaders of state and territorial health agencies. In her role, Kyle leads ASTHO's capacity building and technical assistance portfolio and other organizational strategic initiatives. She has published extensively on the public health workforce, authoring or co-authoring peer-reviewed articles in the *American Journal of Public Health*, the *American Journal of Preventive Medicine*, and the *Journal of Public Health Management and Practice*. She received her master's degree in public health, concentrating in social and behavioral sciences, from the Boston University School of Public Health. Kyle received a bachelor's degree in anthropology from Skidmore College.

Jane Branscomb, MPH, Assistant Project Director at the Georgia Health Policy Center (retired)

Jane Branscomb is retired from the Georgia Health Policy Center at Georgia State University, where she focused on public and private policy levers to drive population health, well-being, and equity. She provided research, training, and technical assistance to local and national clients of the Center and helped groups use system dynamics models and other systems-thinking tools for productive collaboration and strategic decision-making. Jane holds a master's degree in public health from Emory University and a bachelor's degree in engineering from Vanderbilt University.

Ross C. Brownson, PhD, Lipstein Distinguished Professor of Public Health at Washington University in St. Louis

Ross C. Brownson is the Lipstein Distinguished Professor of Public Health at Washington University in St. Louis. He studies the translation of evidence to public health practice and policy, with a content focus on environmental and policy determinants of chronic diseases. Dr. Brownson has authored and/or edited 15 books and over 550 peer-reviewed articles. He has been noted as one of the most productive public health scholars and was named by Thompson Reuters as one of the world's most influential scientific minds.

Dr. Brownson is a former board member of the American Cancer Society, a former president of the National Association of Chronic Disease Directors, and a former president of the American College of Epidemiology. Prior to joining academe, Dr. Brownson was a division director at the Missouri Department of Health.

Edward M. Cahill, MPA, Director of the Fiscal Management Group

Edward M. Cahill began his career in public service through the New York State public management trainee program. He spent 30 years with the New York State Health Department, where he focused on administration and finance. His tenure at the health department culminated in his appointment to director of finance and budgeting. During this time, he served on many joint federal and state task forces dealing with financial issues, as well as committees dealing with local health departments and associations to provide assistance and guidance on public health issues.

In addition to his work with the health department, he supported the work of the Association of State and Territorial Health Officials through its chief financial officers section and as a member of the association's finance committee. He has also been involved in numerous civic and charitable organizations, particularly in finance. After service in the military, he began his career in the private sector in the banking industry, gaining experience in financial analysis and credit extension.

Edward is a graduate of Siena College. He received a Master of Public Administration degree with a concentration in finance from the State University of New York at Albany.

Grace Castillo, MPH, Former Program Associate at the de Beaumont Foundation

Grace Castillo is a former program associate at the de Beaumont Foundation, where she led project management for book publications. She is particularly interested in noncommunicable diseases, global health, and health infrastructure. Previously, Grace worked for the Equity Research and Innovation Center (ERIC) as a student research intern. While at ERIC, she supported a manuscript project documenting a collaborative steering committee's history. She also contributed to a draft guide for researchers interested in beginning community-based participatory research.

Grace graduated from the Yale School of Public Health's Chronic Disease Epidemiology Department with a certificate in regulatory affairs. While completing her MPH degree, Grace interned with the Patient-Centered Outcomes Research Institute, where she worked with the Research Infrastructure team. She earned her BA in English from Yale University.

Brian C. Castrucci, DrPH, MA, President and Chief Executive Officer of the de Beaumont Foundation

Brian C. Castrucci is the president and chief executive officer of the de Beaumont Foundation, which he has built into a leading voice in health philanthropy and public health practice. An award-winning epidemiologist with a decade of experience working in local and state health departments, Brian brings a unique perspective to the philanthropic sector that allows him to shape and implement visionary and practical initiatives and partnerships and to connect research and practice to improve public health.

Brian is also an editor and contributing author to books, including *The Practical Playbook: Public Health and Primary Care Together, Public Health Under Siege: Improving Policy in Turbulent Times, Leading Systems Change in Public Health: A Field Guide for Practitioners*, and *Talking Health: A New Way to Communicate About Public Health*. Brian has published more than 85 articles in the areas of public health systems and services research, maternal and child health, health promotion, and chronic disease prevention. His recent work has focused on the public health needs of large cities, the need for better data systems, and public health system improvements.

Reena B. Chudgar, MPH, Director of Public Health Systems and Services at the Public Health National Center for Innovations at the Public Health Accreditation Board

Reena Chudgar is the director of public health systems and services at the Public Health National Center for Innovations (PHNCI) at the Public Health Accreditation Board, where she leads planning and implementation of PHNCI's portfolio of work. She supports PHNCI's initiatives involving fostering innovation, multi-sector collaboration, public health modernization, and advancing equity.

Reena brings more than 18 years of direct public health experience to her efforts to support health departments and their communities in using innovation as a tool for transformation and to create equitable opportunities for optimal health. She is passionate about social and systems change, addressing root causes of historical and current racial and health inequities, and local and people-centered decision-making. Reena aims to support public health by engaging in dynamic partnerships, fostering cross-sector collaboration, looking to community expertise, and advocating for public health needs.

Prior to joining PHNCI, Reena served as the director for performance improvement at the National Association of County and City Health Officials. She also has experience working internationally in Ghana and Kiribati. Reena received a Master of Public Health degree and a bachelor's degree in chemistry from Emory University.

James E. Dills, MPH, MUP, Senior Research Associate at the Georgia Health Policy Center at Georgia State University

Jimmy Dills is a senior research associate at the Georgia Health Policy Center (GHPC). He works to improve public health by advancing a Health in All Policies perspective on decision-making. His areas of expertise include systems thinking, health impact assessment, and healthy community design. At the GHPC, Jimmy leads several maternal and child health projects, including management of GHPC contributions to the National MCH Workforce Development Center, the National Maternal Health Learning and Innovation Center, and the Maternal Telehealth Access Project. He also leads work on several Health in All Policies projects and provides training and technical assistance to local, state, and national partners related to Health in All Policies.

Jessica Solomon Fisher, MCP, Vice President for Strategic Initiatives at the Public Health Accreditation Board

Jessica Solomon Fisher is the vice president for strategic initiatives at the Public Health Accreditation Board (PHAB). She joined the organization in 2015 as the chief innovations officer of PHAB's Public Health National Center for Innovations (PHNCI). She oversees PHNCI and other strategic initiatives, communications, and education and technical assistance for PHAB. Jessica also helps lead the All In: Data for Community Health collaborative. Previously, she spent 13 years at the National Association of County and City Health Officials, where she served most recently as the senior advisor of public health programs. Jessica earned a master's degree in community planning from the University of Maryland School of Architecture, Planning & Preservation and a Bachelor of Science degree in geography from Ohio University.

Katrina Forrest, JD, Co-Executive Director of CityHealth

Katrina Forrest serves as the co-executive director of CityHealth, working closely with local elected leaders, policy experts, and other key stakeholders to expand the understanding of health beyond healthcare and to drive municipal policy change to expand access to healthy choices and improve the conditions that most influence a person's health.

Before joining CityHealth, Katrina served as both deputy chief of staff and legislative director for former At-Large D.C. Councilmember David Grosso. In that role, she drafted more than fifty pieces of original legislation and was responsible for leveraging community and business relationships to drive the Councilmember's legislative agenda and policy priorities. In 2020 she was the recipient of the Community Champion Award from the District of Columbia Behavioral Health Association for her advocacy on behalf of D.C. residents with mental illness or addictions and for her commitment to advancing behavioral health issues.

Prior to her work in local and state government, Katrina served as a compliance manager with the National Community Reinvestment Coalition, where she worked to eradicate discriminatory practices in housing and banking. Katrina holds a bachelor's degree in Administration of Justice from George Mason University and a law degree from the University of Illinois Chicago John Marshall Law School.

Michael R. Fraser, PhD, MS, CAE, FCPP, Chief Executive Officer of the Association of State and Territorial Health Officials

Michael R. Fraser is the chief executive officer of the Association of State and Territorial Health Officials (ASTHO). ASTHO is the national nonprofit organization representing the public health agencies of the United States, the U.S. territories, and the District of Columbia, as well as the more than 100,000 public health professionals these agencies employ. ASTHO members, the chief health officials of these jurisdictions, are dedicated to formulating and influencing sound public health policy and to ensuring excellence in state-based public health practice.

Michael is the co-author of *Vaccinating America: The Inside Story Behind the Race to Save Lives and End a Pandemic* with Brent Ewig and *A Public Health Guide to Ending the Opioid Epidemic* with Jay Butler. He has also authored many research publications and articles on public health preparedness, infrastructure, and leadership. He is an affiliated faculty member at the George Mason University College of Public Health.

Laura Hanen, MPP, Senior Policy Advisor at Venable LLP

Laura Hanen has more than 25 years of bipartisan experience in government relations and public affairs focused on public health and healthcare policy, advocacy, and communications. She is a member of Venable's legislative and government affairs practice. Laura previously served as a senior vice president at Faegre Drinker's district policy group. She also was the chief of government affairs for the National Association of County and City Health Officials, where she led policy development and federal lobbying for its 2,800 city, county, metropolitan, district, and Tribal health department members. She also served as the director of government relations for the National Alliance of State and Territorial AIDS Directors and senior lobbyist for the American College of Obstetricians and Gynecologists. Laura has a Master of Public Policy degree from Georgetown University and a bachelor's degree from Earlham College.

Shelley Hearne, DrPH, Professor at the Johns Hopkins Bloomberg School of Public Health

Shelley Hearne is a professor at the Johns Hopkins Bloomberg School of Public Health (BSPH), where she brings an extensive track record of leadership, policy impact, institution-building, and teaching in health advocacy to her work. She is BSPH's inaugural Deans Sommer & Klag Professor of the Practice and director of the Lerner Center for Public Health Advocacy. Dr. Hearne is also the executive director of the environmental health philanthropy, Forsythia Foundation. Previously, she was the president of CityHealth, the founder and former executive director of the Trust for America's Health, and the managing director of The Pew Charitable Trusts' health group. Dr. Hearne also led the Big Cities Health Coalition, served as the acting director of New Jersey's pollution prevention program, and was the executive director of the Pew Environmental Health Commission.

Jeannine Herrick, MPH, Founder of Jeannine Herrick Leadership Coaching and Consulting

Jeannine Herrick is the founder of Jeannine Herrick Leadership Coaching and Consulting. She is an adjunct instructor in the Public Health Leadership Department at the University of North Carolina Gillings School of Global Public Health. Jeannine served as the director and leadership coach for the National Program Office for the Emerging Leaders in Public Health initiative. She is a senior member of the Adaptive Leadership Core within the National MCH Workforce Development Center.

Jeannine also supported local and state leaders through her prior role as a senior advisor in training and leadership at the North Carolina Institute for Public Health at the Gillings School of Global Public Health. She has designed and conducted trainings on a variety of topics and provided technical assistance to partners conducting assessments and facilitating strategic planning and change management sessions.

Jeannine has an extensive background in program design and implementation, curriculum development and training, evaluation, strategic planning, partnership development, and donor relations.

Edward L. Hunter, MA, Public Health and Public Policy Consultant

Edward L. Hunter is a public health and public policy consultant, working with clients and partners on strategy, advocacy, research, and evaluation projects. From 2015 to 2018, he was the president and chief executive officer of the de Beaumont Foundation, directing cross-sector partnership, research, data, and policy initiatives to strengthen and transform public health in the United States. Previously, he was the director of the Centers for Disease Control and Prevention's (CDC) Washington Office, where for over a decade he directed the CDC's legislative strategy and was a principal CDC representative to Congress, the presidential administration, and public health organizations. He also served as the associate director of the CDC's National Center for Health Statistics, where he led strategic planning for health information systems and helped policymakers use complex data in policies and programs to improve population health.

William J. Kassler, MD, MPH, Chief Medical Officer at Palantir Technologies

William J. Kassler currently works at Palantir Technologies as the chief medical officer, and before that was the deputy chief health officer at IBM Watson Health. He has spent his career working at the intersection of clinical care and population health: as a health information technology industry executive, practicing primary care internist, epidemiologist, health services researcher, public sector administrator, and health policy expert.

Prior to joining the private sector, Dr. Kassler served as a commissioned officer in the U.S. Public Health Service Commissioned Corps. He started as an Epidemic Intelligence Services officer at the Centers for Disease Control and Prevention (CDC). He later served as the branch chief for health services research and evaluation at the CDC, and then as the senior advisor for health policy in the CDC Washington Office. He was the chief medical officer for the New England Region of the Centers for Medicare and Medicaid Services (CMS), and a founding member in the population health models group at the CMS Innovation Center. Dr. Kassler also served as the state health officer for the New Hampshire Department of Health and Human Services, with leadership roles in public health, social services, and Medicaid.

Dr. Kassler received his MD from the University of Massachusetts Medical School, an MS in nutrition from Case Western Reserve University, and an MPH from the University of California, Berkeley. He completed a primary care internal medicine residency at Brown University and was a Robert Wood Johnson Clinical Scholar at the University of California, San Francisco.

Cynthia D. Lamberth, PhDc, MPH, CLMC, Executive Director of the Kentucky Population Health Institute

Cynthia D. Lamberth is a founding board member and the executive director of the Kentucky Population Health Institute (KPHI). Her work focuses on leadership, communication, environmental health, children's health, and systems change programming and evaluation. Prior to leading KPHI, Cynthia served as faculty and the associate dean for workforce development and community engagement at the University of Kentucky College of Public Health.

Cynthia is also a leadership coach and certified facilitator at ExudeU, a social enterprise focused on inspiring teams and individuals to plan and lead a life they love with greater fulfillment, meaning, and ease. She is the author of books, chapters, and articles on mentoring, leadership, change, and community engagement. A female executive trailblazer with several decades of experience, including being the only woman in the boardroom in her early career, to owning two entrepreneurial businesses, Cynthia brings a sensitivity to equity and inclusion. She has over 30 years of experience, including positions in academia, international consulting, technology, and utility industries, and serves on numerous committees, boards, and community initiatives focusing on equity and improving the lives of all people.

Glenn Landers, ScD, MHA, MBA, Assistant Research Professor in the Andrew Young School of Policy Studies and Director of Health Systems at the Georgia Health Policy Center at Georgia State University

Glenn Landers is an assistant research professor in the Andrew Young School of Policy Studies at Georgia State University and the director of health systems at the university's Georgia Health Policy Center (GHPC). His current portfolio includes the Center's work in rural community health systems development with the Health Resources and Services Administration, the Atlanta Regional Collaboration for Health Improvement, and the Robert Wood Johnson Foundation's Aligning Systems for Health: Health Care + Public Health + Social Services. His portfolio also includes the GHPC's work in long-term services and supports and special projects with the Centers for Disease Control and Prevention and other national partners. Glenn plays a lead role in the GHPC's approach to evaluation and collective impact and its substance use disorder portfolio. His published research has appeared in *The Foundation Review*, the *American Journal of Public Health*, the *Medicare & Medicaid Research Review*, and the *Journal of Health Care for the Poor and Underserved*.

Marissa J. Levine, MD, MPH, FAAFP, Professor of Public Health Practice and Family Medicine and Director of the Center for Leadership in Public Health Practice at the University of South Florida College of Public Health

Marissa J. Levine is the director of the Center for Leadership in Public Health Practice and a professor of public health practice and family medicine at the University of South Florida College of Public Health, where she teaches leadership and focuses on population health improvement. Dr. Levine worked for 16 years in state government, most recently serving as the health commissioner of Virginia and leading the Virginia Department of Health.

As commissioner, Marissa led the creation of Virginia's Plan for Well-Being, an action framework to enhance the conditions for equitable population health and well-being. She is a board-certified family physician with 16 years of experience practicing medicine. She received her MPH from Johns Hopkins Bloomberg School of Public Health and her MD from the Albert Einstein College of Medicine. She completed family practice residency training at the University of Virginia.

Kristen Hassmiller Lich, PhD, Associate Professor at the University of North Carolina Gillings School of Global Public Health

Kristen Hassmiller Lich is an associate professor of health policy and management at the University of North Carolina Gillings School of Global Public Health. She specializes in the application of systems thinking, operations research, and complex systems modeling techniques for health policy and management decision-making. Kristen has worked most extensively in tobacco control, maternal and child health, and mental health system strengthening. Her recent projects involve developing both qualitative and quantitative models that support decision-making to allocate limited resources and translate evidence into real-world practice around stroke care, severe mental illness, and colorectal cancer, in collaboration with state and local partners across the United States.

Robin Matthies, MSW, Director of Public and Behavioral Health Integration at the Association of State and Territorial Health Officials

Robin Matthies is the director of public and behavioral health integration at the Association of State and Territorial Health Officials (ASTHO). Prior to joining ASTHO, Robin was the trauma and resilience program manager at the Wisconsin Department of Health Services' Division of Public Health. One of her areas of interest is how toxic stress in childhood and adolescence contributes to risk behaviors and negative health outcomes. Robin has provided trainings on various health topics and takes a preventative approach when presenting, specifically focusing on resiliency and protective factors. She also volunteers as a crisis counselor for youth who are struggling with suicidal ideation, self-harm, and risk behaviors. Robin received her MSW from the University of Wisconsin–Madison.

Karen J. Minyard, PhD, MN, Chief Executive Officer of the Georgia Health Policy Center at Georgia State University

Karen Minyard is the chief executive officer of the Georgia Health Policy Center (GHPC) at Georgia State University. She has led the GHPC since 2001 and is a research professor with the Department of Public Management and Policy in the Andrew Young School of Policy Studies at Georgia State University. Her research interests include financing and evaluation of health-related social policy programs, with an emphasis on funding mechanisms that enable multisector collaboratives to sustainably finance health and well-being in communities. In addition to overseeing the GHPC's overall strategic vision, Dr. Minyard plays a leadership role in projects that consolidate the center's key learnings from research and practice in the areas of systems thinking, sustainability, and community health systems development.

Carolyn Mullen, Senior Vice President of Government Affairs and Public Relations at the Association of State and Territorial Health Officials

Carolyn Mullen is the senior vice president of government affairs and public relations at the Association of State and Territorial Health Officials, where she leads the federal government relations, public relations, and state health policy teams. Previously, she was the director of government affairs at the American Association for Dental, Oral, and Craniofacial Research (AADOCR), where she developed and implemented its federal policy agenda. Prior to her position at AADOCR, Carolyn was the associate director of health reform implementation and government affairs at the Association of Maternal and Child Health Programs and the associate director of federal affairs for March of Dimes. During her tenure at these organizations, she promoted their federal policy agendas to both Congress and the presidential administration, focusing on appropriations, health reform, and public health policy.

Carolyn is the president of the Coalition for Health Funding board of directors. She was named to the de Beaumont Foundation's inaugural 40 Under 40 in Public Health list, which recognizes leaders whose creativity and innovation are strengthening communities across the country. Carolyn is a graduate of Villanova University.

Jewel Mullen, MD, MPH, Associate Dean for Health Equity at the University of Texas at Austin Dell Medical School

Jewel Mullen is the associate dean for health equity and an associate professor in the departments of population health and internal medicine at the University of Texas at Austin Dell Medical School. She is also the director of health equity for Ascension Seton and the director of health equity and quality at Central Health. Mullen is an internist, epidemiologist, public health physician leader, and the former principal deputy assistant secretary for health in the U.S. Department of Health and Human Services (HHS). While at HHS, she also served as the acting assistant secretary for health and the acting director of the National Vaccine Program Office during the months bridging the transition from the Obama to the Trump administrations. Prior to her work at HHS, Jewel was the commissioner of the Connecticut Department of Public Health.

Jewel's career has spanned clinical, research, teaching, and administrative roles focused on improving the health of all people, especially those who are underserved. Jewel is recognized nationally and internationally as a leader in building effective community-based chronic disease prevention programs and for her commitment to improving individual and population health by strengthening coordination between community, public health, and healthcare systems.

Steve Orton, PhD, Senior Fellow in Public Health Leadership at the North Carolina Institute for Public Health, Core Lead for Change Management at the National MCH Workforce Development Center, and Adjunct Assistant Professor in the Department of Health Policy and Management at the University of North Carolina at Chapel Hill Gillings School of Global Public Health

Steve Orton is an educator who works with leaders and managers in public health organizations to develop skills and to lead organizational change. He is lead author of *Public Health Business Planning: A Practical Guide* and has contributed to collaborative workforce development projects at the University of North Carolina Gillings School of Global Public Health since 1994. He contributed to the Executive Program for Developing Countries; the Management Academy for Public Health; Preventing Violence through Education, Networking and Training (PREVENT); the National Public Health Leadership Institute; the Caribbean Health Leadership Institute; Leadership Novant; and the National MCH Workforce Development Center. What he learns doing leadership work nationally, Steve brings home to North Carolina. He teaches in Gillings' undergraduate degree program in health policy and management and teaches or facilitates Area Health Education Center-sponsored sessions for local public health groups across the state.

Marcus Plescia, MD, MPH, Chief Medical Officer at the Association of State and Territorial Health Officials

Marcus Plescia is the chief medical officer for the Association of State and Territorial Health Officials (ASTHO). He provides medical leadership and expertise across the agency and oversees the association's portfolio of chronic disease prevention and control programs. During the COVID-19 pandemic, he served as ASTHO's principal spokesperson and primary liaison to the Centers for Disease Control and Prevention (CDC).

Dr. Plescia has served in public health leadership roles at the local, state, and federal levels in North Carolina and at the CDC. He has led efforts to enact systemic public health interventions, including expanded cancer screening coverage, prescription drug and disease reporting requirements, revised clinical guidelines, and state and local tobacco policy. He has been prominent in nationwide efforts to transform public health practice to a more population-based, strategic framework, and he led the implementation of the CDC's national colorectal cancer screening program based on this approach.

Dr. Plescia received his MD, MPH, and bachelor's degree from the University of North Carolina at Chapel Hill. He trained in family medicine at Montefiore

Medical Center and is board certified in family medicine. Dr. Plescia has practiced in a variety of settings serving homeless, urban poor, and rural underserved populations. He has published extensively in public health and family medicine literature.

Kris Risley, DrPH, CPCC, Executive Leadership Coach at Kris Risley Coaching

Kris Risley is an executive leadership coach with Kris Risley Coaching. She has served the public health field in this role since being certified with the Co-Active Coaching Institute in 2004. Kris earned her DrPH in maternal and child health from the University of Alabama at Birmingham. She also has a master's degree in developmental psychology.

Kris was a staff and faculty member at the University of Illinois Chicago (UIC) School of Public Health between 2000 and 2018. In these roles, she focused on leadership development of the public health workforce. She worked closely with cross-sector partners to bring a leadership lens to the development of public health practitioners. Kris continued this work as a faculty member with the UIC School of Public Health Doctor in Public Health Leadership Program. In this capacity, she taught a course on personal leadership development for public health practitioners committed to developing skills in systems change leadership.

Kris brings an unapologetic heart to her work with public health professionals, and it is this authentic expression that inspires those she works with to be more, do more, and to have greater meaning and impact in their work and more fulfillment in their lives.

Moriah Robins, MPH, Senior Research Associate at the de Beaumont Foundation

Moriah Robins is a senior research associate at the de Beaumont Foundation. Her focus is on the Public Health Workforce Interests and Needs Survey (PH WINS), the only nationally representative survey of the state and local government workforce. Previously, Moriah served as a research associate on the PHRASES project (Public Health Reaching Across Sectors), a partnership between the de Beaumont Foundation and the Aspen Institute. There she designed and managed the PHRASES Fellows, a program aimed at training public health professionals in framing and communicating the value of public health in a way that resonates with decision makers in other sectors. She earned her MPH in Global Health Program Design, Monitoring, and Evaluation from the Milken Institute School of Public Health at The George Washington University. Moriah holds a BS in chemistry from the University of Maryland in College Park, Maryland.

Sheila B. Savannah, MA, Managing Director at Prevention Institute

Sheila B. Savannah is the managing director at Prevention Institute, where she helps build continuums from local to national efforts to address determinants of health. She is based in Houston and has over 30 years of experience in multisector collaboration and community engagement, with a focus on youth and family involvement to address wellness, safety, and equity. Her work with communities of practice involves using multisector systems transformation to strengthen natural assets and to heal community-level trauma. Sheila leads projects that take a public health approach to improving community environments to address complex issues and co-create solutions for mental well-being, collective trauma, substance misuse, and strengthening community safety. Her team launched a planning initiative in California where five nontraditional collaboratives are receiving technical assistance to prevent domestic and partner violence. She is also working on a project to improve quality of life among children, youth, and families of color in ten communities in the greater Houston area.

Previously, Sheila was a division manager with the Houston Public Health Department and the Office of Adolescent Health and Injury Prevention. She holds a bachelor's degree in journalism from the University of Texas at Austin and a master's degree in psychology from the University of Houston-Clear Lake.

Renata Schiavo, PhD, MA, CCL, Senior Lecturer in Sociomedical Sciences at Columbia University Mailman School of Public Health

Renata Schiavo is a senior lecturer in sociomedical sciences at the Columbia University Mailman School of Public Health's Department of Sociomedical Sciences. She is passionate about health equity and removing barriers that prevent people from leading healthy, productive lives. For over 25 years, Renata has worked at the intersection of public health, global health, health communication, social and behavioral change communication, healthcare, international development, and social innovation. She has worked in the United States, Africa, Latin America, Europe, and Eastern Asia. At Mailman, she has taught courses on society, health equity, and health communication; global trends in child health and development programs; and community-based participatory research. Renata is the author of the internationally acclaimed book *Health Communication: From Theory to Practice*, in its second edition, as well as more than 50 publications and 160 scientific presentations. She also serves as editor-in-chief of the peer-reviewed *Journal of Communication in Healthcare: Strategies, Media, and Engagement in Global Health*; is founder and board president of Health Equity Initiative, a nonprofit membership organization; and is a principal at Strategies for Equity and Communication Impact (SECI), a global consultancy.

Katie Sellers, DrPH, CPH, Senior Advisor for Strategy and Innovation at the Health Resources and Services Administration Maternal and Child Health Bureau

Katie Sellers is the senior advisor for strategy and innovation at the Health Resources and Services Administration (HRSA) Maternal and Child Health Bureau. Prior to joining HRSA in 2021, Dr. Sellers was the executive vice president at the de Beaumont Foundation, where she led the foundation's research and evaluation work, as well as many of the programmatic initiatives. Prior to her time at de Beaumont, Katie served as the senior vice president for science and strategy at the March of Dimes and the chief science and strategy officer at the Association of State and Territorial Health Officials. In both of those roles, Katie led research and evaluation efforts, launched major strategic initiatives, and sought to advance diversity, equity, and inclusion.

Catherine C. Slemp, MD, MPH, Public Health Consultant

Cathy Slemp leads her own public health consulting practice, with current projects focusing on community resiliency and leadership development. From 2018 to 2020, Cathy was the commissioner and state health officer for the West Virginia Department of Health and Human Resources' Bureau for Public Health, overseeing the state's public health activities and partnerships and launching the state's response to COVID-19. From 2002 to 2011, she was West Virginia's state health officer, overseeing immunization programs, outbreak and disease control programs, emergency preparedness and response efforts, and agency quality improvement activities. Concurrently, she served as the state's emergency preparedness director. In this role, she founded and directed preparedness programs, managed multi-million-dollar grants, and led public health agency responses to the 2009 H1N1 pandemic, floods, Hurricane Katrina, 9/11, and other emergencies. Prior to these roles, she was the founding director of the state health department's Division of Infectious Disease Epidemiology and an epidemiologist for the West Virginia Cancer Registry. Throughout her career, Cathy has worked closely with public health agencies, healthcare facilities, and cross-sector partners to build both epidemiology and emergency preparedness infrastructure in communities. Cathy is board certified in public health and preventive medicine and in family practice.

Christina R. Welter, DrPH, MPH, Clinical Associate Professor in the Health Policy and Administration Division, Director of the Doctor in Public Health Leadership Program, and Associate Director of the Policy, Practice, and Prevention Research Center at the University of Illinois Chicago School of Public Health

Christina R. Welter is a clinical associate professor in the division of Health Policy and Administration at the University of Illinois Chicago (UIC) School of Public Health, where she is also the director of the Doctor in Public Health Leadership Program and the associate director of the Policy, Practice, and Prevention Research Center. Christina is a nationally recognized policy practitioner, visionary leader, and practice-based researcher committed to equity-centered policy and systems change. She oversees applied research and workforce development initiatives and has catalyzed award-winning cross-sectoral leadership collaboratives, has co-designed novel capacity-building initiatives, and has built or translated evidence to foster policy adoption and implementation. She co-edited and co-authored *Leading Systems Change in Public Health: A Field Guide for Practitioners*. She received her doctorate in public health leadership from the UIC School of Public Health and her master's degree in public health in health education and behavior from the University of Michigan.

Amber Norris Williams, MS, Senior Vice President for Leadership and Organizational Performance at the Association of State and Territorial Health Officials

Amber Norris Williams is the senior vice president of leadership and organizational performance at the Association of State and Territorial Health Officials, where she provides strategic guidance and direction for member onboarding and engagement, as well as capacity-building and technical assistance services to strengthen and improve state public health leadership and performance, and she leads ASTHO's internal staff development and organizational performance. She has more than 20 years of experience in public health and coalition-building at the local, state, and national levels. She spent more than a decade as the executive director of the Safe States Alliance, a national nonprofit focused on injury and violence prevention. Amber has a Bachelor of Science in education in health promotion and behavior from the University of Georgia and a Master of Science in organizational leadership from Colorado State University, Global Campus.

Introduction to the Strategic Skills Framework

MICHAEL R. FRASER AND BRIAN C. CASTRUCCI

THE TRAINING AND DEVELOPMENT OF public health practitioners is dominated by volumes of information on the technical aspects of public health practice. While this information is vital, there is a lack of real discussion of the cross-cutting strategic skills required for successful leadership and management of public health agencies. If we have learned anything over our careers working in and for governmental public health departments, it is this: the future of public health requires a deep understanding of the specialized, science-based, and technical aspects of what improves health and wellness as well as a broad understanding of the strategic skills that support effective public health practice.

While academic public health training does an excellent job preparing the public health workforce for many of the technical challenges of practice, this book focuses on the political, strategic, and leadership skills that need much more attention in both academic and "on-the-job" training programs for public health professionals. To be successful, contemporary public health practitioners need

Michael R. Fraser and Brian C. Castrucci, *Introduction to the Strategic Skills Framework* In: *Building Strategic Skills for Better Health: A Primer for Public Health Professionals*. Edited by: Michael R. Fraser and Brian C. Castrucci, Oxford University Press. © de Beaumont Foundation 2024. DOI: 10.1093/oso/9780197744604.003.0001 both the scientific knowledge and formal preparation required to be experts in their fields as well as acumen in strategic leadership and management.

We came to this belief along two different avenues. While working in state and local public health agencies, Brian C. Castrucci found that his colleagues included many highly specialized and knowledgeable experts in distinct fields, such as epidemiology, laboratory sciences, chronic disease, and maternal and child health. However, his colleagues' expertise often failed to translate practically into systems change. He realized that public health practitioners—both inside and outside of the governmental public health workforce—need to bolster their existing skills and knowledge with a broader set of skills that support multisector partnership building, improved communication with the public, and increased integration of public health ideas to address the social, political, economic, and community-based determinants of health.

Having worked for national associations of local and state public health leaders, as well as for a brief time in federal service at the Health Resources and Services Administration and the Centers for Disease Control and Prevention, Michael R. Fraser observed the political influences and organizational development challenges to members and colleagues in government that were unrelated to their technical know-how and expertise. These observations led him to further study in leadership, management, and strategy to complement specialized academic training in social science and opened a universe of knowledge about organizational behavior and an evidence-based approach to organizational performance that have been transformative to his leadership of organizations ever since.

Our experiences suggest that the governmental public health workforce should take a more integrative approach to strategic management and technical skills to effectively manage initiatives, engage across sectors, and influence key factors that affect health in communities. Practitioners can develop strategic skills that complement their existing discipline-specific expertise with an ability to gain and apply knowledge from experts in other disciplines, such as transportation, agriculture, and housing. While many of these skills are not unique to public health, they are vital to the sustainability of governmental public health organizations at all levels.

What Are the Strategic Skills?

The process of identifying the strategic skills most critical to the public health workforce began in 2014.[1] Representatives from 31 public health organizations, including discipline-specific member organizations, national organizations, and federal agencies, were interviewed and then convened to identify the cross-cutting priority training needs for the public health workforce over the next decade. The preliminary work laid the foundation for the work that followed.[1] While the initial process articulated strategic skills, those skills were not specifically defined. Also included in the work was a call for the "creation of a convener organization . . . dedicated to workforce development."[2] The de Beaumont Foundation responded by convening the National Consortium for Public Health Workforce Development, which included representatives from 34 national partner organizations, to determine how best to operationalize, promote, and support the transformation of the workforce to include the integration of strategic skills.

The first deliverable from the National Consortium was the release of a report, *Building Skills for a More Strategic Public Health Workforce: A Call to Action.* Using a consensus-building process, the report's authors identified nine indispensable, high-performance workplace skills applicable to the entire public health workforce regardless of specialty or discipline. Since the release of the report, how these skills are defined and operationalized continues to evolve. Figure I.1 provides a list of the strategic skills and their current definitions.

The National Consortium's report also applied the "T-shaped employee" concept to the public health workforce. First proposed in 2015 by Tim Brown, chief executive officer of global design firm IDEO, the idea of a T-shaped employee is one who has deep expertise (the vertical part of the T) as well as cross-functional knowledge (the horizontal piece).[2] The public health workforce includes highly specialized and knowledgeable experts in distinct scientific disciplines (epidemiology, laboratory sciences, chronic disease prevention, injury and violence prevention, and so on) that are the foundation for many

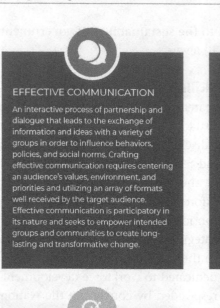

EFFECTIVE COMMUNICATION

An interactive process of partnership and dialogue that leads to the exchange of information and ideas with a variety of groups in order to influence behaviors, policies, and social norms. Crafting effective communication requires centering an audience's values, environment, and priorities and utilizing an array of formats well received by the target audience. Effective communication is participatory in its nature and seeks to empower intended groups and communities to create long-lasting and transformative change.

JUSTICE, EQUITY, DIVERSITY, AND INCLUSION (JEDI)

Advancing JEDI involves an ongoing, intentional effort to create an environment where everyone has a fair opportunity to thrive, enjoy good health, and wholly participate in a full range of life's activities. Supporting JEDI calls for both personal accountability and collaborative group efforts to examine power structures, listen and act on the perspectives and voices of underrepresented/historically marginalized groups, and ensure that all people have real, meaningful access to necessary resources and support systems.

DATA-BASED DECISION MAKING

Encompasses collecting, interpreting, and leveraging data—including "big data"—to identify salient patterns, answer relevant questions, and make effective decisions. The insights generated during data analytics translate into tangible, real-world change and lead to informed actions.

RESOURCE MANAGEMENT

A process through which current and future resources (including finances, staff, individuals with technical or subject expertise, technology, equipment, and any other component integral to organizational or programmatic operations) are strategically and efficiently allocated and deployed to the degree appropriate to achieve organizational and systems-level success and minimize waste.

Figure I.1. Strategic skills for public health: Definitions. Source: Gendelman, Moriah, et al. de Beaumont Foundation, 2021, *Adapting and Aligning Public Health Strategic Skills*, https://debeaumont.org/wp-content/uploads/2021/04/Adapting-and-Aligning-Public-Health-Strategic-Skills.pdf.

disease response efforts illustrative of the vertical part of the T-shaped employee. This expertise alone, however, is inadequate to achieve necessary change to improve the public's health. For public health practice, the T-shaped workforce is one in which there is continued excellence in core scientific disciplines, complemented by strategic skills that allow the workforce to transcend traditional public health disciplines to meet the evolving needs of the public.

CROSS-SECTORAL PARTNERSHIPS
Involves bringing together two or more distinct fields—such as health care and transportation—to yield greater impact and results. Public health professionals skilled in these types of partnerships will be able to foster and sustain meaningful, long-term collaborations that combine a unique set of resources, experience, and knowledge to more effectively and efficiently address complex, multifaceted issues (e.g., the social determinants of health). Public health is expertly positioned to convene these partnerships and help focus their efforts through a public health lens.

SYSTEMS AND STRATEGIC THINKING
A holistic and dynamic understanding of interrelated complex structures—such as public health and health care—as well as the ability to recognize those systems' influences at multiple levels and use those insights to align resources to achieve goals. It involves designing interventions that help people see the overall structures, patterns, and cycles in systems and allows for the identification of solutions that simultaneously leverage improvement throughout the system.

COMMUNITY ENGAGEMENT
Refers to an authentic, mutually beneficial, and collaborative process of working to address issues that affect the health and well-being of particular communities, which often involves prioritizing health equity. Community engagement exists on a spectrum; involves equitable distribution of decision-making power and a focus on community partnering and collaboration; and is rooted in trust and respect.

CHANGE MANAGEMENT
A process to guide individuals, organizations, and systems through the transition from a current state to a desired future state, with an emphasis on learning and resiliency at all levels. Public health professionals skilled in change management will be able to set an example, inspire a shared vision, challenge the status quo, manage uncertainty, and encourage strengths-based action while navigating ongoing challenges to successfully realize needed change.

POLICY ENGAGEMENT
Involves working to inform, influence, implement, and evaluate legislation strategies at federal, state, and local levels in order to leverage long-lasting systems changes to protect and improve the public's health and well-being.

Figure I.1. Continued

State of Strategic Skills in the Governmental Public Health Workforce

Data from the Public Health Workforce Interests and Needs Survey (PH WINS) support the move to elevate the strategic skills in public health practice. First fielded in 2014, PH WINS is the only nationally representative source of data about the governmental public health workforce. It captures individual governmental public health workers' perspectives on key issues, such as workforce engagement, morale, and training needs, as well as emerging concepts in public health and demographic data.

As part of the second PH WINS (undertaken in 2017), participants were asked to assess the importance of several cross-cutting skills and their proficiency with each. Training gaps were defined as areas of high importance but low proficiency. Several of the cross-cutting skills aligned with the strategic skills identified in the National Consortium's report. While not all strategic skills were included in the skills assessed, the top two skills with the most significant training gaps regardless of supervisory level or position in the organization were budgeting and financial management (cited by 55% of participants)—which falls under the Resource Management strategic skill—and systems and strategic thinking (identified by 49% of participants). Other strategic skills with significant training gaps included change management (43%), cultural competency (31%)—part of the Justice, Equity, Diversity, and Inclusion strategic skill—and data for decision-making (28%)—part of the Data-based Decision Making strategic skill. These proficiency assessments underscore the need for continued investment in the development of the skills among the governmental public health workforce.[3] The third PH WINS, fielded in 2021, built on the preceding work by explicitly assessing the presence of the nine strategic skills in order to inform the development of workforce training.[4]

Strategic Skills and COVID-19

We conceptualized this book prior to the emergence of the SARS-CoV-2 (COVID-19) global pandemic, a development that thrust governmental public health agencies and public health management, leadership, and strategy into the spotlight. While our colleagues completed their contributions to the manuscript, COVID-19 continued to rage across the United States and around the globe. We argue that what has been hardest about the prolonged response to COVID-19 in this country is not just the technical or scientific challenges of a global pandemic. Public health professionals have accomplished an amazing amount of work to understand the virus and control it using basic principles of public health science since the virus was first confirmed in the United States on January 21, 2020. For example, while initially delayed, COVID-19 tests were developed and scaled, epidemic containment and mitigation approaches were implemented, interruption of airborne viral transmission has become relatively well understood, and COVID-19 vaccine development has been an unprecedented achievement.

Instead, what has been hardest to professionally witness and in many cases to be part of is the lack of systems thinking and strategic response in our national efforts, including the confusion caused by unclear messaging and public communications about the use of face coverings and physical distancing, the unfortunate politicization of the public health response by many elected leaders and members of the public, the scarcity of data-informed problem-solving and decision-making among some authorities charged with preventing the spread of the virus, and many other examples where strategic skills could have, and should have, been applied. Equally painful is the way that COVID-19 magnified and worsened the disparities and inequities in this country, an outcome that was predictable given prior pandemics and public health emergencies but that has been inadequately addressed in many communities even as of today. A dearth of strategic thinking and leadership, not lack of technical skills and public health science, characterizes our response to this devasting public health crisis. One need only ask; "What is our national COVID-19 exit strategy?" to see that there are competing versions of the way forward, all of which will require significant public health leadership, management, and strategy.

Integrating strategic skills into the governmental public health workforce's existing science-based training will help the nation be more prepared for the next pandemic. For example, through the addition of strategic skills, the public health workforce will be poised to think and strategize across systems to align disparate and competing systems, to efficiently and rapidly pivot and react to changes during future disasters, and to communicate more effectively the nuances of a crisis and justifications for policy decisions. These were precisely the skills needed to enhance our nation's pandemic response. Too often, we presume that strategic skills, like problem-solving, are "learned along the way" or are innate to specific personality types. Instead, like any skill, they are teachable and can be mastered with practice. We believe public health practice can, and will, do better with an integrated approach to workforce development that leverages the best of public health technical expertise and a new and equally significant focus on the cross-cutting strategic skills that promote effective public health practice. Focusing on strategic skills will help public health organizations advance in countless ways.

A Call to Action

The leading recommendations from *Building Skills for a More Strategic Public Health Workforce: A Call to Action* include:

- Elevate strategic skills development to the level of specialized skills.
- Invest in expanding professional development and training in strategic skills.
- Advance the use of strategic skills to support systems instead of silos in public health practice.

This volume seeks to advance these recommendations by defining the nine strategic skills and by providing greater detail, through our contributors' chapters, on each of the skills and why they are essential for public health practice. Ensuring the adoption of strategic skills and training necessary to support their development throughout the public health workforce will require a collective effort across the public health enterprise and governmental public health workforce.

The chapters in this volume highlight leadership, strategic, and management skills and what is currently happening in the field to advance, disseminate, and further these skills in the workforce. Embedding these skills into governmental public health practice will fast-forward the work of public health, moving from disease-focused tertiary services to upstream population health improvements. This book supports and advances the implementation and practice of these strategic skills among public health professionals ready to combine practical information with compelling leadership and management competencies.

We urge training programs and interdisciplinary partners in schools of policy, management, and engineering, as well as professional associations and philanthropy, to build on these chapters to help advance the consortium's recommendations.

We envision this book as a tool for addressing the National Consortium's central criticism of the field of public health workforce development:

> Public health workforce development efforts have remained mired in traditional, disjointed training solutions heavily loaded toward discipline-based content and outmoded approaches. While maintaining excellence in core scientific disciplines continues to be a priority, developers and deliverers of public health education and training need to act in new and different ways if the governmental public health workforce is to gain competency in the strategic skills needed throughout the entire public health workforce.[2]

As stated above, creating these "new and different ways" of building public health workforce competencies in strategic skills should be a priority for academic programs, professional associations, and public health partners nationwide. When we successfully transform the public health workforce to equally balance strategic and scientific skills, we will undoubtedly unlock the full potential of the governmental public health workforce to improve the public's health and create healthier communities.

References

1. Nancy J. Kaufman et al., "Thinking Beyond the Silos: Emerging Priorities in Workforce Development for State and Local Government Public Health Agencies," *Journal of Public Health Management and Practice* 20, no. 6 (2014): 557–565, https://journals.lww.com/jphmp/fulltext/2014/11000/thinking_beyond_the_silos__emerging_priorities_in.1.aspx.
2. National Consortium for Public Health Research Development, *Building Skills for a More Strategic Public Health Workforce: A Call to Action* (de

Beaumont Foundation, 2017), https://debeaumont.org/wp-content/uplo ads/2019/04/Building-Skills-for-a-More-Strategic-Public-Health-Workfo rce.pdf.

3. "PH WINS: 2017 National Findings," de Beaumont Foundation, April 27, 2020, https://debeaumont.org/signup-phwins/explore-the-data/ph-wins-2017-national-findings.

4. "PH WINS 2021 Methods, Dashboard Notes, and Survey Instrument," de Beaumont Foundation, August 3, 2022, https://phwins.org/static/img/ resource_docs/PH_WINS_2021_Instrument_and_Methods.pdf.

1

What PH WINS Tells Us about the Interests, Needs, and Satisfaction of the Public Health Workforce

KATIE SELLERS, MORIAH ROBINS, AND KYLE BOGAERT

WHILE THE GOVERNMENTAL PUBLIC HEALTH agency workforce is essential to ensuring the public's health, few investments have been made to understand dynamics of the public health workforce. The public health literature primarily describes the prevalence or correlates of disease and poor health behaviors aligning with federal research funds. While these investments created a significant knowledge base, as Gebbie et al. wrote in 2002, "Without a competent workforce, a public health agency is as useless as a new hospital with no healthcare workers."[1]

The existing public health workforce literature defined the size and composition of the workforce and identified competencies and training needs. Research conducted by the Centers for Disease Control and Prevention (CDC) and various membership associations have provided critical information on funding and staffing levels, while

Katie Sellers, Moriah Robins, and Kyle Bogaert, *What PH WINS Tells Us about the Interests, Needs, and Satisfaction of the Public Health Workforce* In: *Building Strategic Skills for Better Health: A Primer for Public Health Professionals.* Edited by: Michael R. Fraser and Brian C. Castrucci, Oxford University Press.
© de Beaumont Foundation 2024. DOI: 10.1093/oso/9780197744604.003.0002

individual state and local health agencies conducted their own research to directly identify workforce development needs and potential challenges. Despite the volume of this work, critical gaps existed. Previous public health workforce research focused on specialties in public health rather than the complete workforce. Prior research has also used different methods, time frames, or survey instruments, limiting, if not negating, interstudy comparisons, and it has analyzed data often at the agency level. To effectively monitor the health of the current governmental public health agency workforce, the field needed an individual-level survey that could monitor the health of the workforce and measure insight on current trends that crossed both discipline-specific and state and local organizational silos. In 2014, the Association of State and Territorial Health Officials and the de Beaumont Foundation partnered to create the Public Health Workforce Interests and Needs Survey (PH WINS).

When launched in 2014, PH WINS was the first and only nationally representative survey of individual employees in state and local governmental public health agencies (and that is still true today), and it provides an unprecedented, vital window into the workforce's concerns.[2,3] PH WINS captures the perspectives of the individual staff working in state and local governmental public health agencies on issues such as workforce demographics, engagement and morale, training needs, and emerging concepts in public health. The survey also aims to:

- Help health agencies understand workforce strengths, gaps, and opportunities to improve skills, training, and employee engagement
- Inform and guide future workforce research and development, such as recruitment and retention efforts
- Support the workforce in modernizing traditional public health roles to meet the evolving needs of the public
- Identify demographic trends and their implications for the workforce

Following its first administration in 2014, PH WINS was fielded again in 2017 and 2021, with additional administrations planned for 2024 and 2027. Participating local and state public health agencies could opt for a sample of their staff to take the survey (a subset of participating departments in PH WINS 2014 and 2017 opted for this strategy) or for all staff members to complete the survey (the model for all departments in PH WINS 2021). The 2017 administration included a nationally representative sample of medium-to-large (staff size > 25; population served > 25,000) local public health agency staffs. Because administration was delayed in 2020 due to the COVID-19 pandemic, the 2021 survey included questions measuring public harassment and bullying of the workforce, post-traumatic stress prevalence in the state and local governmental public health agency workforce, impressions of the COVID-19 response, and reactions to the declaration by the CDC that racism is a public health crisis. Results from all PH WINS administrations can be found at www.debeaumont.org/phwins.

The sampling strategy and survey instrument for PH WINS evolved with each administration.[3] PH WINS 2021 recruited all state health agencies (SHAs), all members of the Big Cities Health Coalition (BCHC), and a nationally representative sample of local health departments (LHDs) with a staff size of at least 25 and serving a population of at least 25,000. In addition, all LHDs in Health and Human Services (HHS) Region V (Illinois, Indiana, Michigan, Minnesota, Ohio, and Wisconsin) and Region X (Idaho, Oregon, and Washington) were invited to participate in PH WINS through a pilot program called PH WINS for All. Using employee rosters from each participating health department, 137,446 governmental public health staff nationwide were invited to participate in PH WINS 2021. The survey received 44,732 responses (35% of eligible respondents) representing 47 SHAs, 29 BCHC departments, and 262 LHDs.

State and Local Governmental Public Health Workforce's Knowledge and Expertise

Nationally in 2021, the state and local governmental public health agency workforce is mostly female (79%), non-Hispanic white (54%), and over age 45 (51%). Half of all respondents reported being at their present agency for five or fewer years. Thirty-six percent have five or fewer years of experience in public health practice; 20% have 21 years or more. Thirty-six percent have earned an advanced degree.

Despite a 300% increase in public health graduates since 1992,[4] the proportion of staff with formal public health training remains small, at 14%, and it was unchanged between the 2017 and 2021 PH WINS. The low proportion of public health training in the workforce, coupled with the experience of much of the workforce, both in age and in years of public health practice, means that the workforce may not necessarily have the knowledge and expertise needed to tackle emergent needs of communities. This gap has significant implications for training and workforce development.

Additionally, employee turnover poses a real threat to institutional knowledge in the public health workforce. The potential for significant employee turnover in the state and local government public health workforce due to retirement and other reasons not related to retirement was first identified in the 2017 PH WINS and remains in the 2021 PH WINS. Nearly half (44%) of respondents to PH WINS 2021 said they were considering leaving their organization in the next five years. While this has been similar throughout each fielding of PH WINS, a preliminary analysis comparing employee rosters from 2017 and 2021 shows that actual turnover was two to three times higher in 2021 than it was between 2014 and 2017. The COVID-19 pandemic and its demand on the governmental public health workforce most likely increased intention to leave, with 39% reporting that COVID made them want to leave. Additionally, the proportion of respondents who selected work overload/burnout as a top reason for leaving rose by nearly 20% from PH WINS 2017 to 2021 (24% in 2017 to 41% in 2021). As shown in figure 1.1, the top five reasons for

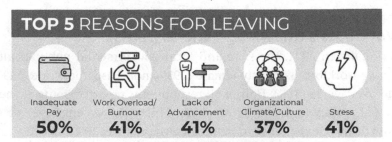

Figure 1.1. Top five reasons for leaving the public health workforce cited in PH WINS 2021. Source: 2021 PH WINS survey data.

leaving cited in PH WINS 2021 were inadequate pay (50%), work over-load/burnout (41%), lack of opportunities for advancement (41%), organizational climate/culture (37%), and stress (37%).

What Are the Training Needs of the Governmental Public Health Workforce?

PH WINS assesses the training needs of the governmental pub-lic health workforce. Between 2014 and 2017, the training needs assessment was revised, based on stakeholder input, to have more specific, actionable skills in the 2017 questionnaire.[3] The section was also restructured into a tiered approach for 2017, survey-ing different skill items according to a respondent's supervisory status.[3] The 2021 PH WINS training needs assessment was updated to align with the refreshed strategic skills released in early 2021.[5] In 2021, the strategic skill domains were: effective communication; data-based decision-making; justice, equity, diversity, and inclusion (JEDI); budget and financial management; systems and strategic thinking; change management; community engagement; cross-sector partnerships; policy engagement; and programmatic expertise. Respondents rated the importance of each item in their day-to-day work as well as their level of competence in performing each skill. Those in the nonsupervisory tier read a basic version of each item, supervisors and managers read a different version, and those in the executive tier read a third, higher-level version. Because employ-ees at all levels self-report their training needs, PH WINS provides managers and leaders with unique insight into opportunities for improvement.

If respondents rated a skill item as having high importance in their day-to-day work but rated themselves as unable to perform or as beginners in that skill, the item was designated a skill gap. The top skill gaps identified in PH WINS 2021 were in the following domains: budget and financial management (54%), systems and stra-tegic thinking (47%), and community engagement (44%). It is impor-tant to note that these top three training needs remained consistent from PH WINS 2017 to PH WINS 2021. The top three training needs are shown in figure 1.2.

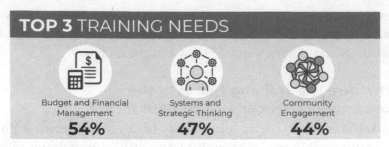

TOP 3 TRAINING NEEDS

Budget and Financial Management	Systems and Strategic Thinking	Community Engagement
54%	**47%**	**44%**

Figure 1.2. Top three training needs cited in PH WINS 2021. Source: 2021 PH WINS survey data.

At supervisory levels, these top three training needs were the same among supervisors and managers. However, nonsupervisory respondents identified their top three training needs as budget and financial management, change management, and systems and strategic thinking. Additionally, executives self-reported their top three training needs as budget and financial management, systems and strategic thinking, and policy engagement.

The consistency in the top training needs from PH WINS 2017 to PH WINS 2021 indicates the need for practical and impactful training in these areas and is part of why this book was written. Furthermore, the differences among training needs for each supervisory level underscore the need to tailor training to meet the specific needs of the various levels of the workforce, in order to be relevant and have the most impact.

We would be remiss if we didn't mention the other strategic skills, because training in those areas is still necessary. Among respondents to PH WINS 2021, 44% need training in change management; 39% in policy engagement; 38% in cross-sector partnerships; 35% in advancing justice, equity, diversity, and inclusion; 29% in data-based decision-making; and 20% in effective communication.

What Is the Future of the State and Local Governmental Public Health Workforce?

The contemporary public health workforce faces a complex landscape and requires a different approach than the public health challenges of the nineteenth and twentieth centuries. Public health in previous eras was driven by infectious disease prevention and treatment and the rising threat of chronic disease, catalyzed by the advent of HIV/AIDS.[6] While the workforce still needs the skills and expertise to combat emergent infectious diseases, as seen with the COVID-19 pandemic, health interventions for the twenty-first century have moved upstream. Frameworks like the HHS's Public Health 3.0 and the CDC's 10 Essential Public Health Services describe a public health infrastructure that addresses the structural factors that affect the health of communities.[6,7] These frameworks have resonated with the field and take public health practice beyond its traditional role. The frameworks advocate for a variety of practices, including robust multisector collaboration and centering equity in public health's work to address the root causes of a community's health.[6,7] To move this forward, managers and leaders must encourage staff to strengthen the cross-cutting strategic skills that help create strong leadership in their workforces.

It is essential to use data to inform and prioritize the workforce development goals and initiatives that will advance the workforce. Recruiting a highly qualified, diverse workforce, ensuring that staff are sufficiently engaged and motivated to remain in their roles, and structuring their agencies to support training and skill development are all complex yet common objectives for leaders and managers. As is true for other types of decision-making, using data (in this case from PH WINS) will guide leaders in creating workforce development initiatives and will provide the rationale for prioritizing certain approaches or focuses.

For example, PH WINS data can be used by leaders to inform their strategies related to employee retention. Insufficient pay heavily influences potential turnover among governmental public health staff, and changes to salary bands are often made systemwide and outside the influence of a single state agency.[8,9] Data from PH WINS reveal other significant factors that can affect staff turnover, such as workplace culture and lack of opportunity for advancement, that an individual leader may be able to change to improve retention.[8] PH WINS data, supported by other national-level research on the importance of employee engagement for retention, can orient managers and leaders to prioritize a positive organizational climate and opportunities for staff advancement—and at low or no cost.

Without relevant data on staff training needs, leaders and managers may be left to rely on anecdotes about both perceived strengths and training deficits. Anecdotal evidence may be misaligned with actual employee needs and hamstring workers' ability to embrace public health's evolving role. By using PH WINS data to prioritize areas for all staff training and development opportunities, leaders and managers can equip staff with the necessary skills for their current roles and current public health practice and can build capacity within the agency for future leaders and future roles for existing staff. As public health becomes increasingly multidisciplinary, it is insufficient to focus on building technical or discipline-specific skills in the workforce. Instead, leaders and managers need to prioritize building the cross-cutting skills of all staff—not just employees working in traditional areas of public health, such as chronic or communicable disease—that are necessary for the future of public health practice.

State and local government agency leaders have demonstrated the value of using PH WINS data to inform their visions for workforce development. For example, one agency designed and launched cross-agency teams to improve employee engagement as a tactic for both recruitment and retention; another used the data as a baseline to build workforce resilience by finding joy in work.[10,11] Other health departments used the data to prioritize and improve internal communication—a critical element of employee engagement squarely in the control of an agency's leadership to address.[12,13] Leaders and managers can also use the data, coupled with information collected from staff, to address systems-level obstacles that may impact employee recruitment and retention.[12,13]

To be effective leaders and managers, public health professionals need to discover what drives their staff, to identify employees' needs and strengths, and to make those factors align with, or contribute to, the agency's vision by fostering and developing a positive organizational climate. Using available data, leaders and managers not only can shape the agency's vision but also can make recommendations for developing the organization they need to address and overcome the complex and lofty challenges in public health. By building cross-cutting and strategic skills in their workforce, leaders and managers can advance their vision and mission to improve population health.

References

1. Kristine Gebbie, Jacqueline Merrill, and Hugh H. Tilson, "The Public Health Workforce," *Health Affairs* 21, no. 6 (2002): 57–67, https://doi.org/10.1377/hlthaff.21.6.57 https://www.healthaffairs.org/doi/10.1377/hlthaff.21.6.57.
2. Katie Sellers et al., "The Public Health Workforce Interests and Needs Survey: The First National Survey of State Health Agency Employees," *Journal of Public Health Management and Practice* 21, Suppl. 6 (2015): S13–S27, https://doi.org/10.1097/PHH.0000000000000331.
3. Jonathon P. Leider et al., "The Methods of PH WINS 2017: Approaches to Refreshing Nationally Representative State-Level Estimates and Creating Nationally Representative Local-Level Estimates of Public Health Workforce Interests and Needs," *Journal of Public Health Management and Practice* 25 (2019): S49–S57, https://doi.org/10.1097/phh.0000000000000900.
4. Jonathon P. Leider et al., "Trends in the Conferral of Graduate Public Health Degrees: A Triangulated Approach," *Public Health Reports* 133, no. 6 (2018): 729–737, https://doi.org/10.1177/0033354918791542.
5. de Beaumont Foundation, "Adapting and Aligning Public Health Strategic Skills," March 2021, https://debeaumont.org/wp-content/uploads/2021/04/Adapting-and-Aligning-Public-Health-Strategic-Skills.pdf.
6. Karen B. DeSalvo et al., "Public Health 3.0: A Call to Action for Public Health to Meet the Challenges of the 21st Century," *Preventing Chronic Disease* 14 (2017): E78, https://doi.org/10.5888/pcd14.170017.
7. Centers for Disease Control and Prevention, "Ten Essential Services of Public Health," 2010, http://www.cdc.gov/nphpsp/essentialServices.html.
8. Kyle Bogaert et al., "Considering Leaving, but Deciding to Stay: A Longitudinal Analysis of Intent to Leave in Public Health," *Journal of Public Health Management and Practice* 25 (2019): S78–S86, https://doi.org/10.1097/phh.0000000000000928.
9. Rivka Liss-Levinson et al., "Loving and Leaving Public Health: Predictors of Intentions to Quit among State Health Agency Workers," *Journal of Public Health Management and Practice* 21 (2015): S91–S101, https://doi.org/10.1097/phh.0000000000000317.
10. Center for State & Local Governmental Excellence, "Innovations in the Health and Human Services Workforce: State and Local Governments

Prepare for the Future," 2019, https://www.slge.org/assets/uplo
ads/2019/11/innovations-in-hhs-workforce.pdf.
11. Kyle Bogaert et al., *Journal of Public Health Management and Practice*,
"Supplement Focus: Public Health Workforce Interests & Needs Survey
2017" 29(1) (2019): S16–S25.
12. Karen McKeown et al., "Using Data to Advance Workforce Development
in Public Health Agencies: Perspectives from State and Local Health
Officials," *Journal of Public Health Management and Practice* 25 (2019):
S180–S182, https://doi.org/10.1097/phh.0000000000000972.
13. Jessica N. Brown, Jonathan Fuchs, and Alexa Ristow, "Prioritizing the
Public Health Workforce: Harnessing PH WINS Data in Local Health
Departments for Workforce Development," *Journal of Public Health
Management and Practice* 25 (2019): S183–S184, https://doi.org/10.1097/
phh.0000000000000975.

Vision, Mission, Strategy, and Culture as Core Concepts of Public Health Practice

MICHAEL R. FRASER

DESCRIPTIONS OF THE CHARACTERISTICS OF high-achieving governmental public health agencies often highlight the agency leader's role as community chief health strategist,[1] a tall order considering some of the obstacles and barriers to implementing strategy in governmental public health practice. For state and local public health leaders to successfully position themselves and their agencies as community chief health strategists, strategy and strategic thinking, not administrative operations, must be their focus. Four core concepts are vital to public health agency leaders who strive to adopt the role of chief health strategist for their agency: strategy, vision, mission, and culture.

Strategy Is about Positioning and Direction-Setting

A goal without a plan is just a wish.
—Anonymous proverb,[2] also attributed to
Antoine de Saint Exupéry

Michael R. Fraser, *Vision, Mission, Strategy, and Culture as Core Concepts of Public Health Practice* In:
Building Strategic Skills for Better Health: A Primer for Public Health Professionals. Edited by: Michael R. Fraser
and Brian C. Castrucci, Oxford University Press. © de Beaumont Foundation 2024.
DOI: 10.1093/oso/9780197744604.003.0003

In the for-profit world, organizations use strategy to describe to investors and shareholders how the company will compete and "win" in the marketplace.[3] In the military, strategy is used to coherently organize the tactical work of winning battles and wars. In sports, strategy is the combination of plays a team will make to try to beat an opponent. Countless volumes describe corporate strategy, and business schools worldwide teach multiple approaches to it. Most contemporary definitions of strategy refer to Harvard Business School professor Michael Porter, whose seminal 1996 article "What Is Strategy?"[4] defines the term as (1) how a corporation creates a unique and valuable position in the marketplace, (2) the trade-offs needed to succeed (what the company will and will not do), and (3) alignment or "fit" among a company's activities.

In governmental public health agencies, the thrust of strategy is similar to corporate strategy: policymakers, partners, and the public require a clear picture of an agency's direction and how it plans to "win." To paint this picture, leaders need to articulate their agency's unique and valuable position, what they will and will not do as an agency to succeed, and how they will achieve fit among the many services the agency offers to the community. Two prior commentaries, "Beyond the Status Quo: 5 Strategic Moves to Position State and Territorial Public Health Agencies for an Uncertain Future"[5] and "The 3 Buckets of Prevention,"[6] are useful primers on the role of strategy and strategic thinking in public health agencies.

In our article "Beyond the Status Quo," my co-author Brian C. Castrucci and I suggest five strategic positions or "moves" governmental public health agencies can make to adapt and evolve for an uncertain future (see figure 2.1). These include: (1) moving from a focus on programs to a focus on populations, (2) moving from clinically driven services to community-wide, population health services, (3) moving from addressing individual patient needs to using policy change for community-wide impact, (4) moving from siloed, "small" data to using enterprise-wide data systems to understand and improve health, and (5) moving toward a rational distribution of public health services based on efficient delivery of community health programs rather than jurisdictional boundaries or geographies. Consideration

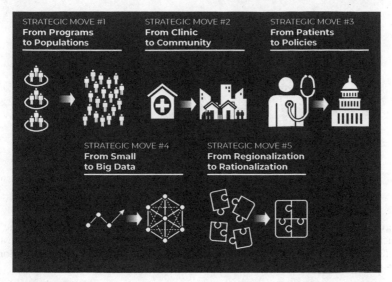

Figure 2.1. Five strategic moves. Source: Fraser, M., & Castrucci, B. C. (2017). Beyond the Status Quo: 5 Strategic Moves to Position State and Territorial Public Health Agencies for an Uncertain Future. *Journal of Public Health Management and Practice:* JPHMP, 23(5), 543–551. https://doi.org/10.1097/PHH.0000000000000 634 Redrawn with permission.

of each of these moves can spur strategic conversations about agency position, trade-offs, and alignment.

In his article "The 3 Buckets of Prevention," John Auerbach presents a strategic framework that practitioners can use to leverage their clinical and community-based work of prevention and health promotion (figure 2.2). These include traditional clinical services, innovative clinical prevention that moves work outside the clinical setting or expands it, and total population or community-wide interventions. Auerbach's discussion of how and why an agency may "play" and "win" in each of these three buckets raises important issues for organizational strategy.

Strategy-setting in government can be challenging, especially when considering the three aspects of strategy Michael Porter describes. The people and communities served by an agency may overlap with other governmental agencies and organizations, and the agency's unique and valuable position vis-à-vis other governmental agencies

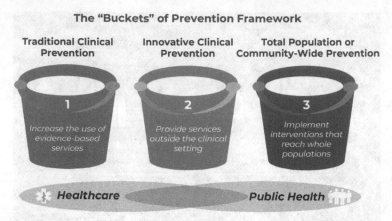

Figure 2.2. Three buckets of prevention. Source: Auerbach J. (2016). The 3 Buckets of Prevention. *Journal of Public Health Management and Practice*: JPHMP, 22(3), 215–218. doi:10.1097/PHH.0000000000000381 Redrawn with permission.

and services therefore needs to be clearly defined and differentiated. Public health's community- and population-wide approach is its biggest asset, but that approach may confound the ability of public health agencies to distinguish their work from the much more visible work of healthcare delivery in a particular jurisdiction.

This problem has led to multiple national initiatives to make the work of public health agencies more visible and understandable to the public. Indeed, there are other agencies that protect and promote the health of the public in a given jurisdiction, such as a state or territorial Medicaid agency or environmental protection agency. A public health agency must therefore either position itself in a way that differs from the others or settle for being confused with them. Agencies that fund or offer both clinical services and population-based prevention activities experience the most trouble with this aspect of strategy: does the agency position itself as a care provider, a primary prevention resource, or a hybrid? How should the agency make tactical moves and winning plays in an environment of constant change and uncertainty in the healthcare sector and a seemingly insatiable demand for clinical services?[7]

Importantly, the resources available to support various activities and programs administered by an agency may be dictated by grants the agency is awarded and the appropriations it receives, and these may or may not closely match the actual needs of a jurisdiction. This challenges alignment, because grant programs and the funding that comes with them do not always fit with agency priorities and strengths. Instead of being based solely on fit, grant programs often are the result of political processes and pressures on policymakers from interest groups and constituents.

As an example, some federal investments in treatment and prevention of opioid use disorder have helped public health agencies to confront the opioid crisis, but they cannot be used to pay for other addiction prevention priorities that are related but not opioid-specific, such as alcohol, nicotine, or stimulant use disorder prevention. Centers for Disease Control and Prevention (CDC) funding to state, territorial, and local health agencies for chronic disease prevention provides an opportunity to address multiple protective factors, such as increased physical activity and nutrition, but health agencies still must align several categorical programs that include asthma, cancer, heart disease, and stroke in their planning and reporting of federal grant activities. In other cases, legislatively mandated initiatives that become strategic imperatives for governmental agencies are not provided with the resources needed to ensure success, resulting in unfunded mandates within programs that can take energy away from strategic priorities and create problems with alignment and fit. No wonder many public health leaders feel more like chief whack-a-mole officers than chief health strategists.

The challenges of working in government complicate agency strategy, adding political, legislative, and regulatory layers to a leader's already difficult tasks of clearly defining an organization's direction and aligning the resources needed to get there. A public health agency's strategic plan should summarize the unique and strategic position leadership wants to take in addressing a jurisdiction's priorities. Agencies without strategy tend to be directionless, characterized by programmatic silos and little cross-agency collaboration. To inspire strategic thinking and collaboration, leaders need to repeatedly share their ideas and efforts to make the multiple activities of an agency fit together and complement one another. Strategy is the foundation for all staff in all positions of the agency. Communicating strategy allows staff to obtain a coherent sense of how their work and their role helps move important goals forward and improves health in their jurisdictions.

A lack of alignment is illustrated in figure 2.3. When adapted to public health, the many arrows represent different functional areas or grant programs in an agency trying to move forward. Alignment and collaboration in such agencies are weak because agency performance is the result of the separate work of specific program areas and not the collective work of the entire enterprise moving toward clearly defined and attainable goals. The leader's goal is to get those arrows all pointing in the same direction.

Absent an agency-wide organizational strategy, programs will likely perform duplicative activities or work at cross-purposes, which may produce friction between parts of the organization. For

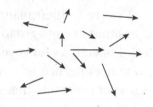

To this:

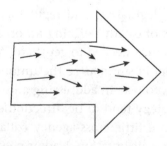

Figure 2.3. Organizational alignment versus lack of organizational alignment. Source: Bregman, Peter. "Execution Is a People Problem, Not a Strategy Problem." *Harvard Business Review*, January 2017, https://hbr.org/2017/01/execution-is-a-peo ple-problem-not-a-strategy-problem. Redrawn with permission.

example, without a comprehensive, agency-wide communicable disease prevention strategy, different approaches may exist for testing and treating HIV than for testing for other viral or sexually transmitted infections/diseases (STIs), even though there may be individuals in the community who are co-infected. These two categorial areas of public health (HIV and STIs) have several funding streams based in two federal agencies (CDC and the Health Resources and Services Administration), different program performance measures, disparate policies supporting each program and how it should operate, and different restrictions on how funding may be used (often to reach the same individual or community), and they may be housed in separate organizational units within the same agency. Strategic thinking about organizational alignment and the fit of these programs within the larger agency can result in a better approach to HIV and STI treatment and prevention and improved outcomes for the community, something currently being promoted by federal and state leaders. Achieving coherence requires team discussions about shared goals and objectives, potentially braiding or blending existing grant programs to complement each other and to reach a common goal, and regular collaboration and information-sharing by staff in these functional areas.

Beyond the Plan: More Strategic Thinking, Less Strategic Planning

In preparing for battle I have always found that plans are useless, but planning is indispensable.[8]

—Dwight D. Eisenhower

Strategic plans are important because documenting goals and measuring progress on key objectives makes strategy known to an organization's leadership and staff. Often, however, the plan itself, as opposed to the process of developing and refreshing it, becomes the defining feature of strategic planning. General Eisenhower's quote suggests that the process of strategic thinking and the process of reaching clarity around an organization's position, its trade-offs, and the fit among programs and services, as well as the resources needed for execution are more important than a plan itself. Rich discussions of where an organization wants to go, which can involve many hours of staff time gathering data about a community's health and the agency's purpose and goals, may result in binders that gather dust on shelves or poster-size summaries that hang in health department break rooms around the country. Developing a plan is an important part, but not the only part, of strategy. As chief health strategists, public health leaders can facilitate dynamic, generative dialogue about where their agency can lead in improving health and can comprehensively forecast and analyze where the health of their jurisdiction is moving.

Strategic thinking and its implementation are described in the excellent case study "Ending Business as Usual" by former Kane County, Illinois, health director Paul Kuehnert.[9] Kuehnert faced a strategic decision about the future of his agency and the community it serves in the wake of a significant funding reduction for agency services: Should the agency continue to provide clinical services that could be performed by other healthcare partners or should the agency reorganize and refocus on supporting the overall health of the community through broad health promotion and prevention work? Through a strategic planning process, the agency's leadership team and county decision makers weighed the trade-offs involved and made the strategic move toward becoming a leaner agency, geared toward protecting and promoting the health of the county and transitioning clinical services to local healthcare partners. The case highlights the importance of strategy, strategic thinking, and the three essential attributes of Porter's definition of strategy: the unique and valuable position of the health department in its jurisdiction, what it will and will not do to succeed, and the alignment among programs and services offered to the community. While the results of the reorganization were acceptable to some and not to others, the strategic conversations about positioning and trade-offs led agency and county leadership to design a plan that allowed the agency to remain solvent amid budgetary constraints and the pressing need for organizational focus.

Mission and Vision: Make Your Cause and Purpose Clear

The only thing worse than being blind is having sight but no vision.[10]

—Helen Keller

There are many ways to define leadership. Donna Petersen, dean of the College of Public Health at the University of South Florida, has noted that her Google search of the term resulted in over 132 million results.[11] In his comprehensive textbook *Leadership: Theory and Practice*, Peter G. Northhouse writes that while scholars have attempted to define leadership for over a century and have reached no consensus, there are essential elements among all interpretations.[12] These include the ability to advance a shared vision and to motivate others to get excited about and support that vision as part of an organizational team.

Leadership often is defined in contrast to management, which is task-based, administrative, and operationally oriented. The job of a leader, as opposed to a manager, is to answer important strategic organizational questions about purpose (*Why are we here?*), communicate about direction (*Where are we going?*), and address questions about motivation (*Why should I go with you?*). Simon Sinek's books *Start with Why*[13] and *Leaders Eat Last*[14] describe how effective leaders must repeatedly communicate an organization's reason for being, what the organization wants to see in the world, and how the organization is going to achieve success both internally and externally, as well as deal with followers' intrinsic and extrinsic needs as individuals agreeing to be led. Answering the vital question about organizational purpose is paramount: purpose informs strategic goal-setting, and strategic goal-setting motivates and engages staff in an agency's work.[15,16]

If the aim of strategy is to lay out an organization's direction and goals, the agency's mission and vision describe the reason or purpose for going there and what agency leadership hopes to obtain as a result. Mission and vision statements are not interchangeable; they are separate concepts. A well-crafted mission statement articulates an agency's unique reason for being and describes what it can do that no other organization can do as well. Management guru Jim Collins's "hedgehog concept"[17] (shown in figure 2.4) can be used to describe the unique combination of factors that define an organization's purpose and activities. Based on a Greek parable about a fox and a hedgehog ("The fox knows many things, but the hedgehog knows one big thing"),[17] the essence of Collins's idea rests at the intersection of three organizational understandings: what the organization is most passionate about, what it can be best in the world at, and what best drives its economic or resource engine. "Great" companies, in Collins's study, used the hedgehog concept to clarify organizational mission and direction; the "good" (but not great) companies he studied had not articulated a hedgehog concept and alignment was scattered, diffuse, or inconsistent.[17] The principle, and the process of reaching the three organizational understandings that underpin it, is a helpful tool for both mission development and overall strategic planning.

Three Circles of the Hedgehog Concept

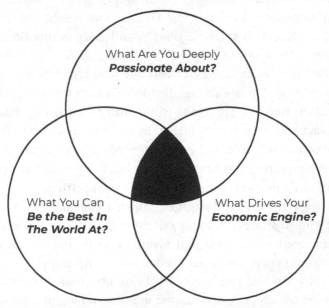

Figure 2.4. The hedgehog concept. Source: Collins, Jim. *Good to Great: Why Some Companies Make the Leap . . . and Others Don't*. Random House Business, 2001. Redrawn with permission.

Effective vision statements are aspirational and describe what an agency wants to see because of its efforts. Vision statements express a desired state that people may find ambitious but is attainable with concerted effort. Visions unite an organization's work around a common cause, but they may be shared by several different organizations with the same aspirations. Vision statements frame an organization's reason for being that transcends individual effort and clearly articulates what the organization stands for. To appropriate from Proverbs: "Where there is no vision, the public health agency may perish."[18] Vision is essential to generating organizational energy and the enthusiasm and motivation needed to carry out an agency's work. Everyone in the organization needs to see how their work contributes to attaining the organization's vision—the leader's job is to make those connections clear and to link vision, mission, and strategy to move the organization forward. This requires constant attention, communication, confirmation, and clarification.

Table 2.1 lists examples of mission and vision statements from two state health agencies and a national public health organization of state and territorial health leaders. The state health agency visions include the aspiration of better health for the entire state. Although that vision might be shared with other healthcare or public health organizations in the same locality (demonstrating that desired futures may be common to several organizations), no other organization has the specific mission of promoting and protecting the overall public health of the entire state. That every-resident reach is unique to the public health agency and defines its mission, differentiating the agency from other public health and healthcare organizations.

The Leader's Role in Creating Organizational Culture

Culture eats strategy for breakfast.[22]

—Attributed to Peter Drucker

Strategy, mission, and vision are vital components of an organization that strives to be its community's chief health strategist. However, without an organizational culture that supports strategic thinking

Table 2.1. Examples of Vision and Mission Statements

Agency	Vision	Mission
Pennsylvania Department of Health	A healthy Pennsylvania for all.	The mission of the Pennsylvania Department of Health is to promote healthy behaviors, prevent injury and disease, and to ensure the safe delivery of quality healthcare for all people in Pennsylvania.
Washington State Department of Health	People in Washington enjoy longer and healthier lives because they live in healthy families and communities.	The Department of Health works with others to protect and improve the health of all people in Washington State.
Association of State and Territorial Health Officials (ASTHO)	State and territorial health agencies advancing health equity and optimal health for all.	ASTHO's mission is to support, equip, and advocate for state and territorial health officials in their work of advancing the public's health and well-being.

Sources: Pennsylvania Department of Health,[19] Washington State Department of Health,[20] and Association of State and Territorial Health Officials (ASTHO).[21]

and that has a clear and coherent mission and vision, an agency will never live up to its strategist role. The most well-crafted strategic plan and most eloquent and inspiring mission and vision statements will fall flat in an organization without a culture that supports effective execution of the plan. Whether or not Peter Drucker ever delivered the phrase, it is a well-known management adage that "culture eats strategy for breakfast."[22]

If an organization does not promote and incentivize alignment and collaboration around shared organizational goals, if its mission and vision statement are unclear or uninspiring, if agency leadership cannot easily articulate the agency's value and contribution to the community it serves, or if the agency lacks a coherent organizational strategy, this culture will lead to suboptimal performance across the agency. Culture, the "way of life" of an agency or "the way we do things around here," drives much of organizational performance and success—the norms and values an agency espouses shape organizational and individual behavior. If an agency promotes collaboration between functional divisions but does not reinforce those behaviors in its organizational culture, employees will not collaborate. If an organization provides training and development experiences in how to effectively collaborate, incentivizes collaboration in its performance review and promotion processes, highlights stories of effective collaboration across the agency, and provides clear expectations about employee collaboration, the agency is likely to succeed. Culture is created across the organization, emerging from both the top and the bottom. It is conveyed to onboarding workers in the subtle ways that staff interact and in the more explicit ways that managers and leaders communicate across the organization.

As described in chapter 1, the Public Health Workforce Interest and Needs Survey (PH WINS), a national survey of the local and state governmental public health workforce, determined that public health practitioners are highly motivated, mission driven, and personally engaged in the work they perform. Employee engagement is high in governmental public health: 93% of PH WINS respondents agreed or strongly agreed that "I am determined to give my best effort at work every day," 94% agreed or strongly agreed that "The work I do is important," and 88% agreed or strongly agreed that "I know how my work relates to the agency's goals and priorities."[23] These responses are good news for strategic leaders seeking to work with highly engaged professionals who understand their organizations' goals and priorities.

PH WINS also includes some cautionary data about workplace engagement and health department culture. This includes findings that less than half of the workforce (46%) agreed or strongly agreed that "creativity and innovation are rewarded" in their agencies, 50% agreed or strongly agreed that "communication between senior leadership and employees is good in my organization," and 56% agreed or strongly agreed that "employees have sufficient training to fully utilize technology needed for their work."[23]

Effective leader communication is vital to making abstract concepts like strategy real to employees. A culture that supports high achievement and performance promotes constructive communication and routinely shares feedback.[15] A culture that invests in workforce training and development is also important, especially for workers who are intrinsically motivated and value professional development and growth at work, as do most public health professionals.[23,24] Creativity and innovation are essential to obtaining organizational results, and organizational culture should use both to address the pressing challenges presented to public health agencies today.[25]

There are several management resources that describe the elements of effective organizational culture.[26] Key features include:

- Clarity of purpose (mission, vision)
- Alignment and collaboration (strategy and shared goals)
- Results and accountability (culture that rewards outcomes)
- Clear values to guide employee behavior that include communication, diversity and inclusion, creativity and innovation, and opportunities for growth and development (norms that guide expected employee behavior and comprise the "way of life" of an agency)

A significant task for public health leaders is to develop organizational cultures that include these features. Culture change can be hard, especially when management and employee relations may be governed by collective bargaining agreements, civil service laws and regulations, and political or bureaucratic processes and barriers. However, leaders can find ways to engage employees and foster cultures that are supportive of agency values even within seemingly rigid and risk-averse bureaucracies. The Association of State and Territorial Health Officials (ASTHO) and the de Beaumont Foundation developed a PH WINS Model Policies and Practices Challenge and collected several examples of successful and transformative workforce development programs in local, state, and territorial public health agencies.[27] These included new performance management systems, policies that promote work–life balance and are supportive of families (such as a "bring your infant to work" program), and agency-specific management and leadership training programs for employees with promotion potential.

Summary

Vision, mission, strategy, and culture are important concepts to explore for public health leaders seeking to assume the mantle of leadership as community chief health strategists. This involves understanding the direction-setting role of strategy and the importance of building a culture to support that direction. Mission and vision are critical to describing an agency's purpose and its aspiration both internally and externally. Clarity of purpose and a vision that unites an agency's diverse functional areas will support not only the leader's role as chief health strategist but also his or her role as chief catalyst for community health improvement.

References

1. "The High Achieving Health Department in 2020," RESOLVE, https://www.resolve.ngo/site-healthleadershipforum/hd2020.htm.
2. Joan Horbiak, *50 Ways to Lose Ten Pounds* (Lincolnwood, IL: Publications International, 1995), 95.
3. A. G. Lafley and Roger L. Martin, *Playing to Win* (Boston, MA: Harvard Business Press, 2013).
4. Michael E. Porter, "What Is Strategy?," *Harvard Business Review* 74, no. 6 (1996): 61, https://hbr.org/1996/11/what-is-strategy.
5. Michael Fraser and Brian C. Castrucci, "Beyond the Status Quo: 5 Strategic Moves to Position State and Territorial Public Health Agencies for an Uncertain Future," *Journal of Public Health Management and Practice* 23, no. 5 (2017): 543–551, https://journals.lww.com/jphmp/fulltext/2017/09000/beyond_the_status_quo__5_strategic_moves_to.19.aspx.
6. John Auerbach, "The 3 Buckets of Prevention," *Journal of Public Health Management and Practice* 22, no. 3 (2016): 215–218, https://www.ncbi.nlm.nih.gov/pmc/articles/PMC5558207/.
7. Peter Bregman, "Execution Is a People Problem, Not a Strategy Problem," *Harvard Business Review* 23, January 4, 2017, https://hbr.org/2017/01/execution-is-a-people-problem-not-a-strategy-problem.
8. "Plans are worthless, but planning is everything," Quote Investigator, https://quoteinvestigator.com/2017/11/18/planning/.
9. Paul L. Kuehnert, "Ending Business as Usual: The Kane County Health Department in a Worsening Fiscal Climate," in *JPHMP's 21 Public Health Case Studies on Policy & Administration*, eds. Llyod F. Novick, Cynthia B. Morrow, and Carole Novick (Netherlands: Wolters Kluwer, 2018), 211–229.
10. "The only thing worse than being blind is having sight but no vision," Philosiblog, https://philosiblog.com/2015/09/03/the-only-thing-worse-than-being-blind-is-having-sight-but-no-vision/.

11. Donna J. Petersen, "Leadership," in *Certified in Public Health: Exam Review Guide*, eds. Karen D. Liller, Jaime A. Corvin, and Hari H. Venkatachalam (Washington, DC: American Public Health Association Press, 2018), 82.
12. Peter G. Northouse, *Leadership: Theory and Practice*, 8th ed. (Los Angeles, CA: SAGE, 2018).
13. Simon Sinek, *Start With Why: How Great Leaders Inspire Everyone to Take Action* (New York: Portfolio, Penguin Books, 2009).
14. Simon Sinek, *Leaders Eat Last: Why Some Teams Pull Together and Others Don't* (New York: Portfolio, Penguin Books, 2017).
15. Gary P. Latham, *Becoming the Evidence-Based Manager*, 2nd ed. (Boston, MA: Nicholas Brealey Publishing, 2018).
16. Sally Blount and Paul Leinwand, "What Is Strategy?," *Harvard Business Review* 74, no. 6 (1996): 132–139, https://hbr.org/1996/11/what-is-strategy.
17. Jim Collins, *Good to Great: Why Some Companies Make the Leap . . . and Others Don't* (London: Random House Business, 2001).
18. Proverbs 29:18.
19. Pennsylvania Department of Health, "About the Department of Health," Pennsylvania Department of Health, https://www.health.pa.gov/About/Pages/About.aspx.
20. "2017–2019 Strategic Plan," Washington State Department of Health, March 2017, https://www.doh.wa.gov/Portals/1/Documents/1200/2017-19%20Strategic%20Plan%20Overview.pdf.
21. "ASTHO Strategic Plan: 2018–2021," Association of State and Territorial Health Officials (ASTHO), https://legacy.astho.org/About/2018-2021-ASTHO-Strategic-Plan/.
22. "Culture eats strategy for breakfast," Quote Investigator, 2017, https://quoteinvestigator.com/2017/05/23/culture-eats/.
23. "PH WINS 2021 Dashboards," de Beaumont Foundation, 2022, https://www.phwins.org/national.
24. Frederick Herzberg, "One More Time: How Do You Motivate Employees?," *Harvard Business Review* 81, no. 1 (2003): 87, https://hbr.org/2003/01/one-more-time-how-do-you-motivate-employees.
25. Rachel Locke, Brian C. Castrucci, Melissa Gambatese, Katie Sellers, and Michael Fraser, "Unleashing the Creativity and Innovation of Our Greatest Resource—The Governmental Public Health Workforce," *Journal of Public Health Management and Practice* 25, suppl. 2 (2019): 96–102, https://pubmed.ncbi.nlm.nih.gov/30720622/.

26. Emma Jeanes, *A Dictionary of Organizational Behaviour* (Oxford University Press, published online 2019), https://www.oxfordreference.com/view/10.1093/acref/9780191843273.001.0001/acref-9780191843273.
27. "de Beaumont & ASTHO Announce Winners of First-Ever PH WINS Challenge," de Beaumont Foundation, September 25, 2017, https://debeaumont.org/news/2017/de-beaumont-astho-announce-winners-of-first-ever-ph-wins-challenge/

Systems Thinking for Public Health Professionals

JANE BRANSCOMB, WITH JAMES E. DILLS, GLENN LANDERS,
KAREN J. MINYARD, AND KRISTEN HASSMILLER LICH

PUBLIC HEALTH PROFESSIONALS UNDERSTAND THAT systems beyond healthcare, such as the law enforcement, criminal justice, education, transportation, and social services systems, powerfully influence population health. Through a confluence of events, 2020 brought into stark relief the realities and consequences of inequities endemic in these systems, with one outcome indicator being the disparate toll of COVID-19 on the Black population. The moment—indeed, the perennial charge of public health—urgently calls for systems thinking.

Concepts and Mindsets

In referring, as above, to the healthcare system, law enforcement system, and education system, we typically mean the components and structures (organizations, agencies, service-delivery protocols, payment policies, etc.) working toward explicit ends. We bound

Jane Branscomb, James E. Dills, Glenn Landers, Karen J. Minyard, and Kristen Hassmiller Lich, *Systems Thinking for Public Health Professionals* In: *Building Strategic Skills for Better Health: A Primer for Public Health Professionals*. Edited by: Michael R. Fraser and Brian C. Castrucci, Oxford University Press.
© de Beaumont Foundation 2024. DOI: 10.1093/oso/9780197744604.003.0004

BOX 3.1. DEFINITIONS OF SYSTEM, SYSTEMS MINDSET, AND SYSTEMS THINKING

System: Interaction components and the structures that govern how they interact to produce certain results over time.

Systems Mindset: Recognition that the observed outcome trend is the result of a system.

Systems Thinking: The skill of accurately discerning the system driving certain results.

---

these systems according to their purported aims; they are silos by definition. (See box 3.1 for definitions of system, systems mindset, and systems thinking.) Yet we know that the causes and solutions to the most stubborn public health challenges are not confined neatly within a single silo.

Systems thinking is about understanding and improving actualities. In this context, we bound systems according to their results; we work to discern the system—the components and structures, regardless of silo—that produces those results. This is the system in which we need to intervene to achieve better outcomes that are sustainable and without unacceptable side effects. We are looking for ways to modify that system's components, structures, or underlying goals, so that the preferred results are its product.

For example, effective, sustainable, systemic solutions to the problems underlying the higher rates of COVID-19 infection, hospitalization, and death among Black individuals do not lie in the healthcare system, even though the concerning metrics are health outcomes. The system we might call the "COVID-19 Black–White disparity system" has roots in inequities in employment, transportation, healthcare access, and other areas. We can make short-term improvements in specific indicators with action in one area, but that approach will only go so far if the other areas go unchanged.

To summarize, a system is a set of interacting components and the structures governing how they interact to produce certain results over time. Components can be all sorts of things, both tangible and abstract, such as people, buildings, knowledge, technology, mindsets, and more. Structures, too, can be tangible or abstract, and include physical arrangements, spatial relationships, stated or implicit rules, policies, and norms. Systems thinking starts with a systems mindset: the recognition that the outcome trend we get is the result of a system in operation. The skill of systems thinking is that of accurately discerning and understanding the system driving certain results.

Systems Thinking

Like any skill, systems thinking exists on a continuum. As largely rational beings, we apply it all the time, with greater or lesser proficiency. We make decisions based on the outcomes we think different options will generate when applied to the system as our knowledge and experience enable us to perceive it. We may become increasingly skillful systems thinkers as we accumulate knowledge and experience, which should lead to better insights and inferences about systems.

Unfortunately, several human characteristics and tendencies interfere. First, our knowledge and experience, especially about complex, population-level processes, are always incomplete. Second, we simply are limited in our ability to hold multiple factors in our heads and mentally play out their complex interactions under various scenarios. Finally, we are prone to human pitfalls like selective memory, confirmation bias, short-term thinking, and overgeneralizing, which limit or distort our individual perceptions.

The good news is that, like many other skills, systems thinking can be strengthened through practice. Below are three reflective prompts that can disrupt the patterns of selective memory and other pitfalls mentioned above. With practice, what begins as deliberate reflection morphs into habit of mind, resulting in greater, internalized skill in systems thinking. In addition, the field of systems thinking offers a variety of useful tools that can help us go beyond our limitations and skirt common cognitive errors to develop more accurate and robust understandings of systems. A few of these are described briefly below, along with four examples from public health practice.

Reflective Prompts

Populations, Not Persons

Systems of concern to public health professionals operate at the population level; causal relationships are on a population scale. For example, while the price of cigarettes may not affect a given individual's behavior, evidence shows that increasing the unit price for tobacco products by 20% would likely reduce the initiation of tobacco use among young people by 8.6%.[1] Price is contributory, not causal, at the level of the individual. At the population level, it has a causal effect. Ask yourself, what is the typical pattern of behavior here? What factors affect the overall trend? Outliers might be informative, but population-level change addresses population-level determinants.

The population in question can be smaller or larger, defined by neighborhood, state, or other geography; by demographic criteria; or by some other commonality. The important point is that a system and its results are considered in aggregate. Which population is in focus? Are there subpopulations within the group that show different trends? Should we address the subpopulation with the most troubling trend to improve overall results while reducing or closing the disparity?

Patterns, Not Points

Point-in-time statistics are one-dimensional. They do not provide much information about a system, and our tendency to infer trends from statistics can lead us to erroneous conclusions and poor decisions. Remembering to consider patterns of behavior over time helps overcome the pitfall of overgeneralizing and provides clues to why a system functions as it does.

Remembering to consider patterns also helps overcome short-term thinking when envisioning likely future results of various decisions today. Are there delays and feedbacks that will cause results to look one way in the near term but another in the longer term—better before worse, or worse before better, for example? Will the results multiply over time, diminish, fluctuate, or level out?

Perspective, Perspective, Perspective

Each of us views a system from our individual vantage point. Our compiled knowledge and experience are incomplete—they are unique to us and thus are valuable pieces of the puzzle, but they are not all the pieces.

Compounding the limitations of our perspective, tendencies like confirmation bias and selective memory can lead us to understandings of a system that are not only incomplete but also distorted. We need, somehow, to see what we are missing and what we are mis-seeing.

There are certain places we can remind ourselves to look. Some components of systems that often go unnoticed are the intangible ones. A factor like trust or morale, for example, can play an essential role in a system even though it might not be easy to quantify. Check for both tangible and intangible, measurable and unmeasurable components and structures in systems. Do not overlook elements that can't be touched or counted if they matter in important ways.

Also, make a point of looking for possible unintended consequences. Did an action with positive results in one area cause unacceptable fallout in another, or could it have? While passenger-side airbags made cars safer for most, they led to an increase in infant deaths in car crashes. The intended fix, moving child seats to the back, also had tragic repercussions: babies were more likely to be forgotten and died due to heat exposure in unattended vehicles. Did, or could, an action yield excellent results overall yet worsen a disparity? There are many innovations that greatly improve health and safety but because of their cost, further widen health disparities based on income and insurance. It is a given that big interventions will have multiple impacts. The more we bring these into focus, the more effective we can be in achieving desired results.

When defining desired results, check the precision and accuracy of the stated or desired goal. Are we discussing the "health system" but actually meaning the "healthcare system"? One is the system that produces the specific health outcomes that exist, while the other is the system that is involved in delivering clinical care to individuals who need it. Do we want our state to have the best health or its best health? If we aim for the former, then our success hinges on other states' health. We "succeed" if theirs is worse than ours, regardless of whether ours has improved or declined.

When it comes to perspective, the most important message is that more is better. We can change our own perspective by viewing a system from different angles. We can remind ourselves to look for intangible components, misaligned goals, and unintended consequences. But the best way to overcome limited perspective is to seek input from others whose perspective is different. Those with different knowledge, roles, experience, and training will surely see something we cannot. Multiple perspectives enable us to see what we are missing—and mis-seeing. The tools below are useful for eliciting, testing, and building on multiple perspectives.

Systems-Thinking Tools

Systems-thinking tools include metaphors, maps, and models that help people visualize and communicate with others about a system's elements, structures, interactions, and results. These tools can bring us closer to understanding the actual system, but they are all simplifications of reality and therefore are not strictly accurate. They are useful to systems thinking by focusing us on populations, patterns, and perspectives. Models go the furthest, mathematically simulating complex interactions that go beyond typical human cognitive limits.

One commonly used metaphor is the iceberg shown in figure 3.1, which illustrates levels of intervention in systems and their relative power in eliciting change. Interventions at the level of structures and mindsets may generate broader and more lasting change than those at the level of behaviors or events, because behaviors and events flow from structures and mindsets. However, interventions at the level of structures and mindsets may be more difficult to bring about or take longer to show results than interventions at the level of events or behaviors. In addition, it is often unconscionable not to respond to events or behaviors. For example, battered women's shelters are not mere Band-Aids; they are crucial, life-saving havens. But they alone cannot solve the societal problem of violence against women, which stems from cultural mindsets and the structures and behaviors they

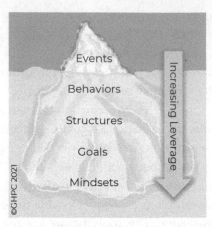

Figure 3.1. The iceberg, a metaphor for levels of intervention leverage in systems. Source: Jane Branscomb/Georgia Health Policy Center, 2021. https://ghpc.gsu. edu/tools-frameworks/systems-thinking/. Redrawn with permission.

produce. So, the iceberg should not suggest that certain intervention types are more or less valuable or important: permanent solutions are likely to require change at many levels. The iceberg is a nudge to look deeply into causes and consider the "systemic-ness"—and thus leverage—of change at various points.

An important type of map, or graphic representation, is the basic trend chart. Groups should study available data for the behavior over time of key variables of interest, which, as noted, can provide clues to the system at work. Figure 3.2 shows an example of a behavior over time chart annotated with factors that influenced the trend at certain points in history. Having team members or stakeholders sketch and share their individual ideas about a trend and its causes also is an excellent way to surface perspectives and move toward deeper, shared understanding.[2]

A stock and flow diagram is another type of system map. Figure 3.3 shows how certain elements in a system move between different states, and factors that influence the rates of movement. This type of map is particularly helpful for identifying time delays and potential buildup or depletion of a variable as well as for considering interventions to alter flows. In this type of simple stock and flow map, open arrows represent pipes through which a stock of something flows

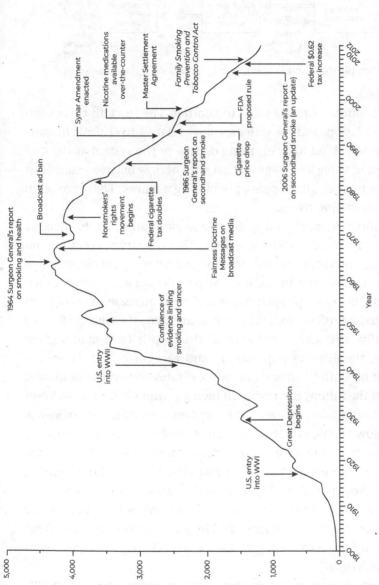

Figure 3.2. Annotated chart of behavior over time: Adult annual per capita cigarette consumption, United States, 1900–2012. Source: National Center for Chronic Disease Prevention and Health Promotion (US) Office on Smoking and Health. *The Health Consequences of Smoking—50 Years of Progress: A Report of the Surgeon General.* Atlanta (GA): Centers for Disease Control and Prevention (US); 2014. Figure 2.1. Adult (≥ 18) per capita cigarette consumption and major smoking and health events, United States, 1900–2012. Available from: https://www.ncbi.nlm.nih.gov/books/NBK294310/figure/ch2.f1/.

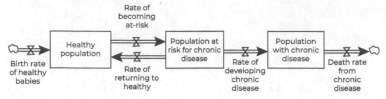

Figure 3.3. Simple stock and flow map. Image courtesy of Jane Branscomb.

from one condition or state (box) to another. The stock in this example is a population, and the states are ones relative to chronic disease. Cloud symbols stand for everything outside of the system as the user has defined it. Valve icons signify that rates of flow between states can decrease or increase, like opening or closing a faucet. These are often the target of interventions.

For example, prenatal care policies and programs aim to increase low-risk births and decrease high-risk births. Obesity prevention and remediation interventions aim to slow the rates of development of risk factors for diabetes in the low-risk population and diabetes incidence in the high-risk population, as well as to increase the flow from high-risk to low-risk status. Diabetes management strategies influence the mortality rate. One way to "read" the map is to look at a given stock—say, the diabetes population—and recognize that its level is dependent on both its inflow and outflow rates. When the outflow is lower than the inflow, the stock will increase, and vice versa. To lower the diabetic population over time requires lowering the incidence rate to below the death rate. Doing this gradually reduces not only the human toll of disease but the investment required for disease management. Simple stock and flow maps like this—or more complex ones—can help partners see where their various efforts come into play; the synergies among their efforts and how all are part of the puzzle; where there may be gaps; and in general, how an "upstream" solution can have a cascading influence in reducing multiple downstream challenges.

Following are four examples that describe additional applications of systems thinking and systems-thinking tools.

Shifting Mindsets and Policies Through Health Impact Assessment

JAMES E. DILLS

Health impact assessment (HIA) is a tool that can support multiple strategic skills. HIA is a framework that puts systems thinking into practice with the cross-sector stakeholders needed to influence social determinants of health and equity. Beginning in 2013, the Georgia Health Policy Center successfully used HIA to catalyze collaboration between public health and affordable housing stakeholders, shifting mindsets and informing policy changes around housing as a platform for population health and wellness.

The HIA of state-level affordable housing policy recommended three revisions to better promote health among residents of new or renovated affordable housing units and surrounding communities. The first was to integrate geospatial data about public health risk factors into the siting criteria used by the state housing finance authority. This would confer a more nuanced understanding of community contexts and the types of affordable housing features that could best promote well-being in them. The second revision was to incorporate school-quality scores into siting incentives. This would give children in affordable housing access to better schools. The third revision was to align design standards with existing best practices for healthy community design, for the benefit of residents and neighbors alike.

A range of housing-sector stakeholders participated in studying these issues, developing new appreciation for health and housing as interconnected components of a community system that also includes education, transportation, and other sectors. HIA created an action-oriented, evidence-informed space for the diverse stakeholders to collaboratively explore potential policy changes.

The results have contributed to improved opportunities for health among over 10,000 low-income households since initial policy changes took effect in 2015. Further, the collaboration and associated mindset shifts led to ongoing cross-sector collaborations that continue to shed light on interrelationships between housing and health in Georgia.

Causal Loop Mapping in Developmental Evaluation

GLENN LANDERS

Efforts to collaborate on collective community change can be highly complex and can be impacted by multiple factors both within and beyond the control of partners. Causal loop mapping can help to unravel the web of factors influencing a given effort's success and provide leaders with actionable insights.

In this example, a developmental evaluation of a collective impact initiative launched by the Colorado Health Foundation entailed reviewing multiple data sources—meeting minutes, emails, direct observation notes, and group progress reports—for recurring patterns of group behavior. The aim was to identify productive or counterproductive patterns, thereby offering the collective impact collaborative opportunities to adapt, alter, or end a particular approach.[3]

The map in figure 3.4 emerged from evaluators' review of data. Collaborative members, in this case, were enthusiastic about the process: When new data and information were presented that touched on their process or goals, they characteristically responded with positive spirits, morale, and energy. At times, however, the new and energizing

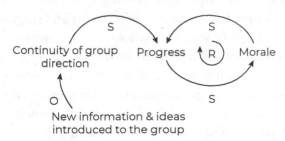

Figure 3.4. Causal loop example: Colorado Health Foundation. Changing direction can lead to a downward spiral of progress and morale. Arrows show causal relationships between the factor at the tail and the one at the head. S denotes the same direction: an increase in A results in an increase in B, or a decrease in A means a decrease in B. O denotes the opposite direction: an increase in A means a decrease in B, or a decrease in A means an increase in B. The R inside the circular arrow denotes a reinforcing loop. This suggests either a vicious cycle (if you don't like the direction of change) or a virtuous cycle (if you do like the direction of change). Source: Jane Branscomb/Georgia Health Policy Center, internal analysis of data.

48

information shifted the group's focus instead of reinforcing the direction they had previously set. In these instances, new input reduced the continuity of the group's direction, which in turn disrupted their progress. This set up a negative reinforcing loop, where lower morale further impeded action and progress.

When evaluators shared the simple map illustrating this dynamic, the group recognized the counterproductive pattern they had not before been able to see. This new awareness led them to seek ways to avoid being sidetracked by new information if it did not reinforce the direction they had chosen for their work.

Cultivating Systems Thinking and Informing Policy through Modeling
KAREN J. MINYARD

For 12 years, the Georgia Health Policy Center has worked with Georgia legislators to build their systems-thinking skills. Those interested in leading their chambers' health policy deliberations spend 24 contact hours in Health Policy Institutes learning about health, healthcare financing, access, system dynamics, and conversational capacity. While each cohort is small, a tipping point of over 20% of each chamber's members have now received certificates. This creates the environment for deeper, systemic examination of policy issues.

While many systems-thinking tools are useful for legislative policy analysis, one of the most impactful is a system dynamics (SD) model, which quantifies system relationships depicted by maps, using the best available evidence to support computer simulation of future trends likely to result from selected interventions.

The first SD model used for policy in Georgia focused on childhood obesity. It was built collaboratively with a group of legislators, legislative staff, and experts in nutrition, physical activity, epidemiology, economics, and system dynamics. Legislators specified policy options for inclusion that they considered possible to implement, and data from published literature and content experts were used to build out the model. The result was a credible tool that stimulated rigorous discussion about policy options for curbing childhood obesity in Georgia.[4]

In the subsequent legislative session, institute participants' deepened understanding contributed to the passage of Georgia's Student Health and Physical Education (SHAPE) Act, which launched a collaborative effort to address issues of childhood obesity. The model was refined as more research and data emerged, contributing to continuation of the SHAPE Act when it was due to sunset.[5]

Now executive and legislative branch leaders in Georgia accept SD models as effective tools to support health-policy decision-making. Their requests have led to development of additional models, one addressing low birth weight, which was used in Georgia's Planning for Healthy Babies 1115 waiver application, and another addressing injury prevention.[6] In 2020, Health Policy Institute participants raised maternal mortality as a priority. The process of mapping the challenge with them was launched, with a goal of building a model for use in examining upcoming policy options.

Focusing Partnerships with System Support Maps

KRISTEN HASSMILLER LICH

Public health professionals' role in facilitating impactful stakeholder collaborations relies heavily on multiple strategic skills. Systems thinking is particularly important in convening partners with diverse knowledge and perspectives, who may be coming from different organizations, disciplines, and even sectors. System support mapping (SSM) is a structured group activity that helps partners build clarity around their own and each other's responsibilities and needs within a shared scope of work.[7]

Participants in an SSM exercise start with a set of concentric circles on a large sheet of paper. In the inner circle they write a one-to-four-word label for their role in the initiative being studied. In the surrounding circle they add their responsibilities or activities supporting the initiative. Next, they list their most critical needs for accomplishing each responsibility. In the final circle, they name specific resources they currently use to meet each responsibility. Participants reflect on how well the available resources support their work. Once responsibilities, needs, and resources are mapped in detail, participants are

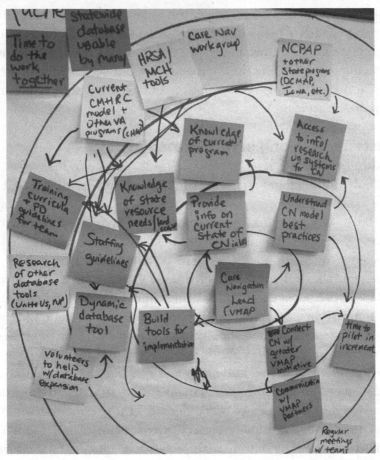

Figure 3.5. Example of system support mapping. Photo courtesy of Kristen Hassmiller Lich.

asked to note outside the largest circle the important wishes they have for being better supported (see figure 3.5).

The National Maternal and Child Health Workforce Development Center at the University of North Carolina uses SSM with state and territorial Maternal and Child Health Block Grant (Title V)-led teams working on collaborative initiatives. When SSM is used early in collaborations, it helps partners to share what they want or feel best positioned to bring to the team, and it helps to clarify hopes and expectations for members of sometimes poorly defined, budding initiatives. For more established initiatives, SSM maps illuminate changes needed to better support the system of responsibilities under way. SSM can also be used to document current collaboration systems, to facilitate transferring the approach from one setting to another or to plan for sustaining a collaboration amid change, such as funding or partner turnover.

Systems Thinking in the Strategic Skills Framework

Systems thinking and strategic thinking are intrinsically linked to one another and are important to the rest of the identified strategic skills. Systems thinking is essential in effectively addressing the deeply embedded mindsets, structures, and behaviors underlying challenges of justice, equity, diversity, and inclusion. Furthermore, as illustrated above, many systems-thinking tools are helpful in putting data into perspective, communicating complex issues, and engaging community members and partners across different backgrounds and sectors. The iceberg metaphor situates policy as a structural factor in systems, affirming its importance as a leverage point. Finally, systems thinking is key to leaders' strategic management of resources and change. Cultivating our systems-thinking skills—recognizing that systems cause observed outcomes, discerning those systems incisively, and using tools and prompts to avoid cognitive limitations and pitfalls—is a lifelong venture with professional and personal returns.

References

1. Community Preventive Services Task Force (CPSTF), *Reducing Tobacco Use and Secondhand Smoke Exposure: Interventions to Increase the Unit Price for Tobacco Products* (CPSTF Finding and Rationale Statement, last updated May 21, 2014; Atlanta, GA: CDC, 2014).
2. Larissa Calancie et al., "Using Behavior over Time Graphs to Spur Systems Thinking among Public Health Practitioners," *Preventing Chronic Disease* 15 (2018), https://www.cdc.gov/pcd/issues/2018/17_0254.htm.
3. Glenn Landers, Kelci Price, and Karen Minyard, "Developmental Evaluation of a Collective Impact Initiative: Insights for Foundations," *The Foundation Review* 10, no. 2 (2018): 10, https://scholarworks.gvsu.edu/tfr/vol10/iss2/10/.

4. Karen J. Minyard et al., "Using Systems Thinking in State Health Policymaking: An Educational Initiative," *Health Systems (Basingstoke, England)* 3, no. 2 (2014): 117–123, https://pubmed.ncbi.nlm.nih.gov/25013722/.
5. Kenneth E. Powell et al., "Systems Thinking and Simulation Modeling to Inform Childhood Obesity Policy and Practice," *Public Health Reports* 132, suppl. 2 (2017): 33–38, https://pubmed.ncbi.nlm.nih.gov/29136493/.
6. Rachel Ferencik and Karen Minyard, "Systems Thinking in Injury Prevention: An Innovative Model for Informing State and Local Policies," *The Western Journal of Emergency Medicine* 12, no. 3 (2011): 273–274, https://www.ncbi.nlm.nih.gov/pmc/articles/PMC3117600/.
7. Larissa Calancie et al., "System Support Mapping: A Novel Systems Thinking Tool Applied to Assess the Needs of Maternal and Child Health Title V Professionals and Their Partners," *Journal of Public Health Management and Practice* 26, no. 4 (2020): E42–E53, https://pubmed.ncbi.nlm.nih.gov/30807460/.

Change Leadership

The Opportunity for a Renewed Public Health Vision

CHRISTINA R. WELTER, KRIS RISLEY, CYNTHIA D. LAMBERTH,
JEANNINE HERRICK, AND STEVE ORTON

Introduction

Change leadership in public health is needed now more than ever. Even before the COVID-19 pandemic, public health practitioners faced multiple simultaneous and diverse challenges that required new knowledge, skill sets, and approaches to address population health improvement and health equity. Whether addressing long-term issues, such as chronic diseases and behaviors or mental health, emerging threats like the opioid crisis, or ongoing issues like preventing food-borne outbreaks, public health practitioners must develop new capacities to organize a response and to mobilize others to address whatever issues are at hand. The COVID-19 pandemic exacerbated this need and required practitioners to respond from a place of inadequate infrastructure to mount the largest public health response in history.

Christina R. Welter, Kris Risley, Cynthia D. Lamberth, Jeannine Herrick, and Steve Orton, *Change Leadership* In: *Building Strategic Skills for Better Health: A Primer for Public Health Professionals*. Edited by: Michael R. Fraser and Brian C. Castrucci, Oxford University Press. © de Beaumont Foundation 2024. DOI: 10.1093/oso/9780197744604.003.0005

Successful change leadership is more likely if we use change frameworks and processes and internalize positive concepts and principles about change. This chapter and chapter 5 discuss and present an approach for leading change. This chapter looks at the nature of change today, articulates processes for addressing change from a leadership level, and describes how cultivation of leadership practices and development of leadership skills are needed at the individual and interpersonal levels to facilitate an effective change process.

The Nature of Change in Public Health Today

Public health's mission has always been to improve health, and in so doing, to address major health challenges. Public health's twentieth-century successes, such as improvements in workplace and motor vehicle safety, resulted in a 25-year increase in life expectancy.[1] Many of these successes overcame challenges that required technical or subject matter expertise and that could be solved with complicated but concrete solutions.

Health improvement today, however, is particularly thorny. While the challenges of the past have not gone away, public health agencies and their partners now also face greater problems. Today's public health challenges are more complex than ever before; they have no simple, single solution. No one person or organization can address issues like climate change. Instead, multiple sectors with diverse expertise will need to work over time to make an impact.

These complex challenges come at a time of overall disinvestment in public health. Governmental public health has experienced major workforce reductions due to retirements and lack of funding, resulting in a loss of expertise and knowledge about how public health works. The 2017 Public Health Workforce Interests and Needs Survey (PH WINS), for example, reported an increase in state government employees' intentions to retire in the next five years.[2] Recent data suggest that the state workforce now numbers 94,000, down from over 108,000 in 2008, and local health departments (LHDs) are down to 153,000 staff from 184,000.[3] As a result, many health departments lack historical and institutional memory, and they lack support for mission-critical positions.

Further, the COVID-19 pandemic has illuminated and exacerbated long-standing, profound, and terrible health and economic disparities that are the result of generations of structural racism. Black, Latinx, and Indigenous people are more likely to be hospitalized or die from COVID-19.[4] Reasons for these extreme disparities in health outcomes include centuries of inequity in education, income, employment, housing, and access to healthcare. These health inequities require systems-level changes that those working in public health must address.

Public health practitioners are being asked to transform, and to be more versatile in, their ability to respond to a variety of issues and at a pace faster than before. They are also being asked to develop new skills to help facilitate large-scale systems change, and to do more with less. Thus, practitioners must be prepared to gather, assess, and mobilize diverse cross-sector partners and communities to respond to the ever-changing environment in innovative ways. Such transformation requires a focus on the development of the individuals and teams in our workforce so they feel supported in growing toward their strengths and evolving in their leadership capacity in ways they may not have anticipated. Change is not easy, but leaders can help lead the way.

Why Is Change So Difficult, and How Can You Increase Adaptation Capacity?

Change challenges all of us. It requires you to alter your mindset, your behaviors, and your patterns of living and working. Typically, when you are asked to make a change of any kind, it takes time, persistent effort, and trial and error to adapt your expectations and approaches from the old way of doing things to the new way. In leading change, the goal is to help increase your own and your colleagues' and partners' readiness and adaptation capacity so that collectively we can successfully make change transitions. There are a few things to keep in mind as those of us in public health consider leading change.

First, for most people, the benefits of a change must be compelling enough to outweigh the costs. Most of us need clarity about what is personally expected to alter the way we live or work, and we must have the mental, emotional, and physical capacity to make the change. In a simple example, think of a time when you or a loved one might have wanted to make a change to improve eating habits, to increase exercise, or to get more sleep. To make such a change, you needed information about healthy ways of living, the resources and flexibility to make those changes (e.g., healthy food or access to safe places to walk), and emotional support from peers. Even then, the change was difficult to make because old habits die hard. Unfortunately, some people experience multiple heart attacks or a disease diagnosis like diabetes before they change their behavior, and some do not make changes even after experiencing severe health challenges.

Second, leading change requires pacing the expected shift. When change happens at all levels of your life (i.e., personally, at work, and within society), occurs too fast and simultaneously, is not what you expected, or came without education about ways to adapt to or to address the change, this is known as future shock. Future shock makes us unable to adjust to a change. Instead, we resist, and the change initiative may fail. Initiatives promoting change readiness help individuals and organizations increase their capacity and develop resilience in the face of change. These initiatives help to pace change in ways that individuals can understand it, address it, and make the change.

Third, leading change requires being able to adapt and learn as you go. You prevent resistance to change and the possibility that a change initiative will fail by increasing your adaptation capacity. Adaptation capacity is the amount of energy that individuals and teams need to understand and address the change desired.[5] The goal is to implement change management and leadership strategies that promote learning, so that people understand the change, connect to the change personally, and see ways in which they personally and collectively can adapt to the change under way. This is not about forcing people to like the change, but about helping them see how their strengths may be used, albeit differently than before, to address and learn the new way.

A Renewed Vision: Creating an Adaptive Workforce of Change Leaders

The vision for public health should be not just about creating healthy people in healthy communities. To address today's complex challenges, public health professionals also need healthy work environments that foster learning and growth. You must constantly grow, learn, ask questions, and build new skills to generate innovative and meaningful approaches to community challenges. You have an opportunity for a renewed vision: creating an adaptive workforce capable of change leadership to take on today's complex challenges.

To address the kinds of changes we see today in public health, we propose an adaptive leadership framework. According to Heiftz, Linsky, and Grashow (2009), *adaptive leadership* is the practice of mobilizing people to tackle tough challenges and thrive.[6] In the adaptive leadership model, leadership is not about hierarchies, titles, or decisions being made primarily by people in positions of authority. Rather, leadership is a process that involves the active contribution of the knowledge and skills of all people at all levels. This is a big mindset shift for public health practitioners, especially those working in governmental public health, where leadership is viewed primarily as hierarchical and exercised by those in positions of authority.

If an organization uses the adaptive leadership model, it increases its likelihood of developing resilient leaders, teams, organizations, and communities because it builds the capacity of the entire workforce and not just those in leadership positions. Successful adaptive leadership is reflected in organizations that create a workplace culture focused on growth through learning from one another about successes and failures and then adapting as needed. The learning-and-growth mindset makes staff members increasingly ready for change and helps them build the capacity to lead it.

To realize this renewed vision, it is helpful to have a process and key concepts to follow. For the process, there are a few steps you can take to build an adaptive workforce for leading change; the steps are outlined in table 4.1. Following them can launch the development of personal and interpersonal leadership.

Table 4.1. Steps to Change Leadership Using an Adaptive Approach

Step	Description
Step 1. Practice systems thinking and understand the context	• Understand the strengths, challenges, opportunities, and threats at the ground level and at the systems level, internally and externally
Step 2. Define the change and its scope	• Identify questions to consider about the type, scope, and approach to change based on the environmental context
Step 3. Plan your change process	• Define the current state, the future state, and how you will get there • Prepare to repeat this process to address complex change • Set up the process to promote learning
Step 4. Build capacity for your success	• Build emotional intelligence, set vision and values, apply a clear strategy, and communicate with and engage the workforce
Step 5. Develop your workforce to build a learning organization to lead change	• Understand how to build individual, team, and organizational adaptation capacity

Steps to a Change Process Using an Adaptive Leadership Model

Step 1. Practice Systems Thinking and Understand the Context

A critical first step in practicing adaptive leadership to lead change is to understand complex problems. Complex problems require you to deeply examine what might be causing the problem as well as the diverse ways in which a problem can be addressed. To create this understanding, adaptive leadership requires systems thinking. Systems thinking allows leaders to see the forest and the trees in order to identify the underlying structures generating change.[6] One systems thinking approach to understanding complex challenges is to conduct an environmental scan. An environmental scan is a systems-thinking tool that can be utilized to collect program development data both to look at and for information on points of alignment or divergence between what capacity you have to do the work versus external demands and opportunities. In a SWOT or SWOC analysis, the situation is explored for strengths, weaknesses, opportunities, and threats/challenges. To understand the context of the change, use interviews, website or document reviews, and other literature to help inform yourself about what is going on.

Step 2. Define the Change and Its Scope
The second step in a change process is to define the problem and the change that you intend to address. There is no one-size-fits-all definition of change or process to achieve change; rather, deciding on the change process depends on the type of change you want to see. There are several questions to consider about types, scope, and approach to consider as you plan for change:

- What kind of challenge exists? What is the need for the change?
- How significant is the change, and how fast does it need to occur?
- Who needs to be involved, and what is the level of their involvement?
- What do you want to see that is different because of making a change?

In the adaptive leadership model, there are two types of challenges: technical and adaptive. Technical challenges have more straightforward answers, a solution that is evident and can be addressed with existing knowledge, and a situation that does not change. An example is addressing budget cuts. While this is not an easy task, there are likely reasonably known revenue and costs that can be evaluated, and approaches to address resource distribution. Technical challenges generally can be solved in a straightforward, linear, and cause-and-effect fashion—and often (although not always) can be solved in a relatively short amount of time.

An adaptive challenge is complex. The situation often changes, requiring leaders to constantly monitor the problem and likely change response approaches; there are many opinions about the cause of the problem; there is no one solution (many experts and many solutions are needed to fully address the challenge); and making an impact takes decades or more. Adaptive challenges often require a diverse group of experts collaborating over time, learning together in iterative, ongoing cycles. An example of an adaptive challenge is climate change. There are multiple political, environmental, and economic forces causing climate change as well as differing perspectives about the cause and solutions; no one individual, national, or even global solution will solve the problem. It will take decades of collaborative, multilevel, and diverse approaches to reverse its effects.

Step 3. Plan Your Change Process

With a systems-thinking lens and an adaptive challenge, you can begin your change process. It is useful to consider how the adaptive leadership change process will occur—where do you start, where are you going, and how do you get there? Kurt Lewin proposed one of the most widely used change models in the United States—one that identifies the current state, the transition state, and the future state.[7] The current state helps to describe the strengths, opportunities, and challenges to reaching the future state. The future state describes the vision of where we want to head next, what the organization might look like, and how it might operate. The transition state is the messy time, when expectations and roles may not be clear, people are struggling to make the desired change, and resistance is most likely.

Because few adaptive and complex challenges are linear, iterative cycles of learning are required. The adaptive leadership model of change includes a cycle of learning and reflection to observe, interpret, intervene, and repeat. As we plan, we know that with complex challenges, change will not occur overnight. We need multiple cycles of learning.

Step 4. Build Capacity for Your Success

The goal of a change process in the adaptive leadership model is to create a learning organization. A learning organization is one that has a learning culture supported by leadership that promotes knowledge, skills, and application of the following: generative ideas, systems thinking, inquiry, and challenges to mental models or deeply held beliefs or ways of thinking. Building capacity to promote learning requires a few key elements.

First, you need to improve your own and your team's emotional intelligence. This includes providing opportunities to build self-awareness through setting a personal vision, grounding the work in personal values, and building personal mastery. This also includes building social awareness and relationship management, such as having empathy and compassion for others' perspectives and world views.[8] Second, you need to create a clear and compelling shared vision of the future. A vision is a profound statement that presents an emotional connection to a desired future and presents a clear picture of where individuals, teams, and organizations should direct their energy.[9] Third, it is important to establish shared, explicit values that everyone is personally passionate about, that they can apply to their work to create motivation and commitment, and that can be used to guide decision-making.[10] Fourth, you need to develop and apply a common strategy and approach to the work that will guide you and your team to reach the vision; this also helps to balance organizational capacity with community needs.[11] Fifth, fostering regular communication, engagement, and workforce development is crucial. Sharing ongoing information that clarifies why the change is happening, what is occurring, and how it is occurring helps people manage expectations and understand the impetus for change.[12] In addition, a learning organization will have organizational spaces and structures for sharing feedback and promoting dialogue and learning through meetings, workshops, and conversations to build team cohesion and acceptance.[13]

Step 5. Develop Your Workforce to Build a Learning Organization to Lead Change

The goal in adaptive leadership is to increase resilient leaders, teams, organizations, and communities; increase learning capacity to understand and address change; and design and address complex problems more effectively and with less effort. You want to increase your readiness for change and ability to adapt more easily by helping individuals address their challenges in reaching the future state at a pace and approach that uses their strengths. In short, you want to create a learning organization. A learning organization is one that excels because it is flexible, adaptive, and productive in situations of rapid change.

To create a learning organization, it is important to understand how you can develop an adaptive leader. An adaptive leadership approach moves beyond the provision of a set of trainings that support positional and technical leadership. Instead, it uses a developmental approach to leadership that applies a learning process and growth mindset to ever-changing challenges. Development occurs in the adaptive leadership approach in three ways:

1. Individuals develop and grow in their abilities to lead change over time, regardless of their position in the organization.
2. Leadership development occurs at multiple levels in an interactive way—at the personal, team, organization, and community levels.
3. Leadership development takes time. While learning must happen at all levels, there is no one right place to begin, and learning is a lifelong process. You can begin at the personal, team, or organizational level.

To encourage learning, we begin with a focus on personal leadership development.

Leading Change Begins with Personal Leadership

Personal leadership in public health addresses practitioners' interest, willingness, and capacity to learn about themselves and to lead their lives in meaningful and impactful ways consistent with who they are and that empower them to create desired changes. Just as every change initiative must have vision, strategy, communication, trust, and a focus on learning, leaders must be clear about their values, vision, strategy for achieving that vision, and structure for continuing to learn about themselves as leaders, and they must be part of a culture that fosters leadership growth. While a focus on personal leadership development is not sufficient to lead successful change efforts, it is a necessary but often neglected component of leadership development that affects our ability to lead change effectively.

Personal leadership is important to leading change for two reasons. First, having a strong sense of personal values and vision helps you stay engaged in your work and provides clear guideposts for how you can best lead change. If you're not clear about why you do the work you do, it is hard to compel others to collaborate on your vision. Many public health leaders are committed to their work because it is mission driven. It is easy, however, to get caught up in the day-to-day bureaucracy and lose sight of why we do what we do. It is not uncommon to forget our passion or even why we got involved in public health work in the first place. As a result, we may feel frustrated, perform poorly, burn out, and even switch roles or quit our job altogether.

Second, personal leadership is important because it gives us permission to engage in lifelong learning and to have compassion for others who also are always learning. Armed with this awareness, you can be an adaptive leader with greater capacity to truly hear others' perspectives and ideas. Without this humility, you may be overly confident that your perspective is the right one and therefore not be open to other approaches. You lose an opportunity to learn from unique perspectives and new ideas. With increased self-awareness and self-confidence, you have greater capacity to appreciate that each of us is likely to have a piece of the puzzle that can move us forward together.

At a basic level, having a strong sense of emotional intelligence is the foundation for personal leadership. Goleman, Boyatzis, and McKee define emotional intelligence as the capacity to be in tune with ourselves and with others.[8] It includes two primary competencies, each with two components: (1) personal competence, including self-awareness and self-management, and (2) social competence, including social awareness and relationship management.

On Developing Personal Competence as a Leader

Personal competence involves building self-awareness and self-management skills. The self-awareness component includes being attuned to your inner self, aware of your leadership strengths and gaps, and having confidence in yourself as a leader.[8] The self-management component involves having self-control, being adaptable and achievement-focused, taking initiative, and being optimistic.[8] You can begin to develop personal competence by articulating your values or guiding principles and personal vision, as well as by being aware of, and managing, the emotions or self-doubt that will most certainly arise while leading a change effort. Articulating your values is a good place to begin.[8]

In their book *Resonant Leadership*,[14] authors Boyatis and McKee offer a straightforward exercise to help readers articulate a core set of values. In their exercise, you select your top 15 values and then narrow down the list to your top five values, which you rank in order of importance. In Brené Brown's book *Dare to Lead,* she recommends a maximum of two core values, stating, "Our values should be so crystalized in our minds, so infallible, so precise and clear and unassailable, that they don't feel like a choice—they are simply a definition of who we are in our lives."[15] Many leaders choose to explore their values with the guidance of a leadership coach. Working with a coach helps you to harvest a rich set of values that you might not otherwise be able to identify on your own. Clear values become a compass to inform the development of your purpose (i.e., calling) and public health vision. Armed with these three foundational elements of personal leadership—values, purpose, and public health vision—you likely will feel more confident in your ability to make decisions that lead to successful change efforts.

As an example, a seasoned local public health leader undertook a values clarification exercise and identified social justice as her primary value. While this is not an uncommon value in public health, her ability to explicitly articulate this as a core value based on prior experiences in her life provided her with a level of clarity about what professional efforts she would undertake to support this value, as well as which efforts were less of a priority. Tying her decision-making to a specific value gave her a level of confidence that she had not felt in her role until then. Prior to having this focus, she felt overwhelmed by her work, paralyzed about making decisions, and lacking in confidence about her ability to achieve the vision she aspired to in her community. The process of identifying her core values also provided her with the confidence she needed to elevate her role and take on higher-level responsibilities. As a result, she was in a better position to make greater change.

Articulating a shared vision is necessary in any change effort. To create a shared vision, it is helpful for you first to be clear about your personal vision. A personal vision may reveal itself through the clarification of your values. Explicitly articulating a personal vision keeps us grounded and focused, which is particularly helpful during challenging times. Similarly, building commitment toward a shared vision keeps everyone motivated, especially when change is challenging. Kouzes and Posner describe a process for getting to a shared vision: (1) articulate your values, (2) look at current trends and important topics of conversation, and (3) imagine a desired future (personal vision).[16] From this place, listen deeply to others to determine what matters to them and where their visions intersect with, or add to, your vision.

One public health professional was ready to leave her job because she felt like she was the wrong fit for the work. She undertook a values and vision clarification process and developed a calling as well as a vision statement. This process inspired her to declare her commitment to making her vision a reality. She defined her calling as mobilizing and engaging communities to have an urgency to act and to achieve greater good across race, religion, gender, geography, social status, and sexuality. She envisioned a world where every person has access to the resources needed—in a sustainable fashion—to achieve their full potential. To work toward this calling and vision, she committed to creating time and space to talk across fences to collectively identify issues and root causes, and to have a place at the communal table where change can be planned and achieved by working from the ground up and the top down. This process grounded her in her work, gave her renewed commitment, and bolstered her confidence. It also inspired her partners to want to work more closely with her.

In the process of developing personal leadership, you must address self-doubt, a very human experience that can impede our ability to lead change efforts. Self-doubt can be heightened by high-risk change initiatives. This experience is also known as imposter syndrome and exists in most people even in the absence of evidence to support one's doubts.

It is important to identify self-doubt and to determine strategies to address it. Self-doubt usually means feeling like you are "not enough," or that you are "too much." Developing personal competence will assist in your efforts to address any self-doubt. Rick Carson's book *Taming Your Gremlin: A Surprisingly Simple Method for Getting Out of Your Own Way* is one useful resource for overcoming self-doubt.[17] A public health professional who believed she was not smart enough to lead a new project was able to identify a set of on-point action steps when she reflected on the following question: "If you were smart enough to lead this new project, what would you do?" Acting "as if" gave her permission to identify a set of steps she would take to get the project off the ground. As it turned out, she was smart enough to lead this new project; her self-doubt was unnecessarily holding her back.

These strategies for developing personal competence as a leader will help you determine your own unique leadership and learning opportunities. If articulating values or vision is a challenge for you, that is a good place to start. If you have significant self-doubt even in the presence of much success, that may be your starting place. For others, identifying your leadership strengths is the best place to start to determine how best to lead a change effort.

On Developing Social Competence as a Leader

Putting personal values, vision, and awareness of strengths to work in interpersonal relationships is the everyday application of leadership. Goleman, Boyatzis, and McKee[8] call this building social competence. Social competence involves building social awareness and relationship management skills. The social awareness component involves building empathy, organizational awareness, and service. The relationship management component involves building our ability to inspire, influence, manage conflict, work as a team, develop others, and serve as a catalyst for change. Strong interpersonal skills allow you to develop effective relationships with others, which increases the likelihood your work together will have greater impact.[8]

Obtaining competence in relationships requires you to reflect on your own and others' world views and how your biases may affect what you want to accomplish with others. These biases and assumptions are referred to as mental models, or strongly held beliefs, or ways of thinking that can either enhance or impede communication.[6] Mental models determine what you see, how you see, and how your thoughts form and lead to behaviors. Every person gives meaning to observations and bases actions on them. Being open to the reality of a range of mental models gives perspective and understanding about potential barriers to successful communication and accomplishments.

A model for addressing conversations (and examining assumptions as well as self-protective tendencies) is the Ladder of Inference.[18] The Ladder of Inference describes how mental models are unconsciously formed. The Ladder of Inference consists of seven steps, with the reasoning process starting at the bottom of the ladder.[18] People select facts from events, which they interpret from prior experiences. The interpreted facts form the basis for assumptions, which in turn lead to certain conclusions. Then a person proceeds to act based on what may be very wrong assumptions or inferences. For example, a staff member takes an idea to her manager. The manager responds that this is an interesting idea. The employee first makes an inference—because the manager gazed out the window and looked at her phone before answering, maybe she doesn't value the suggestion. Next, the employee infers that the manager doesn't think the idea is responsive, or doable, because she used the word "interesting." After that, the employee decides that the manager doesn't really value her ideas and stops making suggestions. In contrast, an effective adaptive leader with strong relationship management creates a communication climate with staff where negative inferences rarely proliferate because the team is confident in their roles and trusts the team and the manager.

There are specific tools you can use to gain insight into developing emotional intelligence. These tools go a long way in helping you develop your personal leadership capacity. The insights gained assist in crafting a personal plan of action for developing personal

Table 4.2. Assessment Tools to Build a Personal Leadership Plan for Leading Adaptive Challenges

Assessment Tool	Purpose
Emotional Intelligence 2.0[1]	Assesses your emotional intelligence
Strengths Finder 2.0[2]	Identifies your top strengths
Strengths-Based Leadership[3]	Identifies your strengths aligned with leadership domains
Emergenetics (Atlanta, GA and New York, NY respectively)[4]	Identifies your thinking and behavioral preferences for approaching work and life
Myers Briggs Type Indicator[5]	Identifies your personality characteristics and how you operate effectively and ineffectively with each
DiSC (Dominance, Influence, Steadiness, and Conscientiousness)[6]	Measures your work style on noted characteristics and how to build better work relationships based on this style
Enneagram (Atlanta, GA and New York, NY respectively)[7]	Identifies your personality type
Change Style Indicator[8]	Identifies your preferences for the pace and type of change
Communication Style Indicator[9]	Identifies your communication style and preferences based on your personality type

[1] T. Bradberry and J. Greaves, Emotional Intelligence 2.0 (San Diego, CA: TalentSmart, 2009).
[2] T. Rath, *Strengths Finder 2.0* (New York: Gallup Press, 2007).
[3] T. Rath and B. Conchie, *Strengths-Based Leadership: Great Leaders, Teams, and Why People Follow* (New York: Gallup Press, 2008).
[4] G. Browning, *Emergenetics (R): Tap into the New Science of Success* (Harper Collins, 2010).
[5] I. B. Myers, *The Myers-Briggs Type Indicator: Manual* (1962).
[6] https://www.everythingdisc.com/.
[7] D. R. Riso and R. Hudson, *Understanding the Enneagram: The Practical Guide to Personality Types* (Houghton Mifflin Harcourt, 2000).
[8] https://storefront.mhs.com/collections/csi.
[9] https://cst-tap.com/.

leadership as well as your unique approach to adaptive leadership. See table 4.2 for a list of personal leadership assessment tools.

Emotional intelligence in the form of personal and social competence is critical for promoting innovation and creating opportunities for a new vision for public health. Putting emotional intelligence into play through the articulation of personal values, vision, and awareness of strengths, along with social intelligence vis-à-vis cultural sensitivity, openness to diverse opinions, and service to communities, provide the opportunity to create long-lasting, meaningful change.

Summary

This chapter describes the challenge of change in public health and the need for adaptive leadership, a process for mobilizing diverse groups to lead complex change and thrive. This framework is increasingly being adopted in public health as a relevant approach for practitioners looking to build a skill set and a practice in leading change. The chapter concludes by exploring personal leadership and ways to develop a personal leadership foundation to lead change and weather the challenges associated with the process.

References

1. "Ten Great Public Health Achievements—United States, 1900–1999," *Morbidity and Mortality Weekly Report* 48, no. 12 (1999): 241–243, https://www.cdc.gov/mmwr/preview/mmwrhtml/00056796.htm.
2. Kyle Bogaert et al., "Changes in the State Governmental Public Health Workforce: 2014-2017," *Journal of Public Health Management and Practice* 25, suppl. 2 (2019): S58–S66, https://journals.lww.com/jphmp/fullt ext/2019/03001/changes_in_the_state_governmental_public_health.10. aspx.
3. Jonathon P. Leider, "New Workforce Estimates Show Public Health Never Recovered from the Great Recession. Then Came COVID-19," *Journal of Public Health Management and Practice Direct,* May 20, 2020, https://jphm pdirect.com/2020/05/20/new-workforce-estimates-show-public-health-never-recovered-from-the-great-recession-then-came-covid-19/.
4. "Covid-19: Introduction to COVID-19 Racial and Ethnic Health Disparities," Centers for Disease Control and Prevention, December 10, 2020, https://www.cdc.gov/coronavirus/2019-ncov/community/health-equity/racial-ethnic-disparities/index.html.
5. Ronald A. Heifetz, Alexander Grashow, and Marty Linsky, *The Practice of Adaptive Leadership: Tools and Tactics for Changing Your Organization and the World* (New York: Harvard Business Press, 2009).
6. Peter Sengue, *The Fifth Discipline Fieldbook: Strategies and Tools for Building a Learning Organization* (New York: Currency, 2014).

7. Kurt Lewin, "Frontiers in Group Dynamics: II. Channels of Group Life; Social Planning and Action Research," *Human Relations* 1, no. 2 (1947): 143–153, https://journals.sagepub.com/doi/10.1177/001872674700100 201.

8. Daniel Goleman, Richard Boyatzis, and Annie McKee, *Primal Leadership: Unleashing the Power of Emotional Intelligence* (New York: Harvard Business Press, 2013).

9. Jim Collins and Jerry I. Porras, "Building Your Company's Vision," *Harvard Business Review* 74, no. 5 (1996): 65, https://hbr.org/1996/09/building-your-companys-vision.

10. Patrick M. Lencioni, "Make Your Values Mean Something," *Harvard Business Review* 80, no. 7 (2002): 113–117, https://hbr.org/2002/07/make-your-values-mean-something.

11. Michael E. Porter, "The Five Competitive Forces That Shape Strategy," *Harvard Business Review* 86, no. 1 (2008): 78, https://hbr.org/2008/01/the-five-competitive-forces-that-shape-strategy.

12. John P. Kotter, "Leading Change: Why Transformation Efforts Fail," *Harvard Business Review* 73, no. 3 (1995), https://hbr.org/1995/05/leading-change-why-transformation-efforts-fail-2.

13. Patrick Lencioni, *Death by Meeting: A Leadership Fable . . . About Solving the Most Painful Problem in Business* (Hoboken, NJ: John Wiley and Sons, 2010).

14. Richard E. Boyatzis and Annie McKee, *Resonant Leadership: Renewing Yourself and Connecting with Others Through Mindfulness, Hope, and Compassion* (New York: Harvard Business Press, 2005).

15. Brené Brown, *Dare to Lead: Brave Work. Tough Conversations. Whole Hearts.* (New York: Random House, 2018), 189.

16. James M. Kouzes and Barry Z. Posner, *The Leadership Challenge*, 3rd ed. (San Francisco, CA: Jossey-Bass, 2003).

17. Rick Carson, *Taming Your Gremlin: A Surprisingly Simple Method for Getting Out of Your Own Way*, rev. ed. (New York: William Morrow Paperbacks, 2008).

18. Chris Argyris, *Intervention Theory and Method: A Behavioral Science View* (Reading, MA: Addison-Wesley, 1970).

Leading Change at the Team and Organizational Levels

.JEANNINE HERRICK, CHRISTINA R. WELTER, AND STEVE ORTON

IN CHAPTER 2, FRASER INTRODUCES FORMER Kane County, Illinois, health director Paul Kuehnert, who had to make tough choices about strategic moves for his agency. Although Kuehnert's organization made painful cuts to preserve the department, eliminating positions and reducing the nonpersonnel components of budgets to zero, it was ultimately unsuccessful: the department closed and started over. Kane County is a valuable case study because its situation is familiar to people in governmental public health: a forced reimagining of the role a public health agency should play amid budget pressures and rapid change in the healthcare and public health environments.

We have worked extensively with state and local public health agencies that are imagining new roles for themselves. Their visions are leading them to expand their capacity in order to execute innovative strategies for changing their communities. In this chapter, we draw primarily from our experiences teaching and coaching Maternal and Child Health Block Grant (Title V)-funded teams in the

Jeannine Herrick, Christina R. Welter, and Steve Orton, *Leading Change at the Team and Organizational Levels* In: *Building Strategic Skills for Better Health: A Primer for Public Health Professionals*. Edited by: Michael R. Fraser and Brian C. Castrucci, Oxford University Press. © de Beaumont Foundation 2024. DOI: 10.1093/oso/9780197744604.003.0006

National Maternal and Child Health Workforce Development Center, and as staff members of the National Program Office of the Kresge-sponsored Emerging Leaders in Public Health (ELPH) program. This chapter shares lessons from our work with these forward-thinking agencies and leaders.

One of the agencies in the ELPH program is in Lubbock, Texas, and its story offers a sequel to the Kane County case study. Elected officials in Lubbock announced in 2011 that they would close the public health agency and outsource mandated functions,[1] primarily because the agency had lost some grant funding and officials wanted to put the building to a different use. A community campaign (and a food-borne outbreak) ultimately preserved the department, but it had to be largely rebuilt.

In 2019, two leaders from this small health department began working toward a new role: acting as a navigational hub. The agency would facilitate a comprehensive, systems approach for residents utilizing myriad healthcare and social services. Through extensive partnership-building, the agency repositioned itself. When the local managed care substance abuse program was threatened with closure, the health department was able to step in and continue managing it—and build in prevention-focused efforts. When a rare outbreak of Verona integron–encoded metallo-β-lactamase-producing carbapenem-resistant *Pseudomonas aeruginosa* (VIM-CRPA) occurred, the agency helped broker extensive CDC-provided technical assistance in a way that kept the healthcare community cooperative and supportive. The community, including municipal leaders, in turn rallied around the health department during COVID-19 response efforts with extensive volunteerism and support for prevention measures.

The future is bright, with an expanded staff and increased annual budget, and intentional efforts to center equity are taking hold in city institutions. Plans for public health infrastructure improvements include a new community-centered building. Lubbock's COVID-19 vaccination efforts have been well represented in local, state, and national media. The agency has become an integral leading voice in the community.

This chapter is for and about people who experience the same need to adapt in the face of changing circumstances. The steps include seeing what is changing (which might require new ways and directions to look), getting comfortable with not knowing what to do for a time (which may require new ways of leading), developing a series of guesses about what will work next (which may require testing and new tolerance for mistakes), and then slowly moving forward on a path on which only the first few steps are clear (which may require courage). We see common factors in agencies managing these changes well: emotional intelligence, conversational capacity, problem-solving skills, and the humility to ask authentic questions and listen.

Understanding the Why: Building Buy-in

Organizational and community transformation is strictly a team sport. Your organizational change results will depend on a team's facilitating and communicating a process. Your change process team might include formal and informal leaders eager to engage. A balanced group with varying strengths will keep things moving. A clear plan for the change process creates a sense of stability and intentionality and will reassure those who prefer change in small increments. Key responsibilities of the group include: establishing communication channels, developing a central repository for staff support (such as trainings), supporting change agents, establishing a decision-making structure, creating evaluation structures (timelines, task tracking, performance objectives and review), and celebrating successes, loudly and broadly.

Adaptive change requires deep focus. Your organizational change rationale must be made crystal clear to all members of the organization. Leaders as change agents must share examples of how your change can increase the value of the work that staff members do and explain how it can reliably improve outcomes.

Our ELPH program participants from the Rhode Island Department of Health provide an example. When the state public health agency started communicating about its transformational new role—to advance social justice in all aspects of its programs and services—leaders carefully built the messaging around themes from listening sessions and town halls. Change agents helped share the news about why the change was called for and what the hoped-for outcomes would be. The "new role" message got a positive reception from staff, who were eager to engage in a new way forward, and through conversation, some of the anticipated resistance was muted.

Change leaders provide multiple opportunities for staff to discuss why change is, or will be, happening. You want staff to feel clarity at this stage, because subsequent stages will be more challenging and less well defined. If you transform job roles, some staff may leave to do the work they personally value. Others will stay but will want time to grieve the loss of something that is changing (a beloved program, a cherished clinical role). Expect these responses and support both groups.

We highlight an example from maternal and child health: Florida's Children's Medical Services leadership planned and then announced that they would enhance their managed care plan functions (including case management) by contracting with a vendor. Strategic investments in workforce development ensured that staff who wanted to continue in case management could move to the vendor agency. The change team then focused on transforming the remaining workforce to oversight and strategist-related roles. The team piloted, created new training, and built system supports for the staff who stayed in order to develop systems-thinking capacity. These actions resulted in new multisector relationships and networks, facilitated referral in those networks, and created new roles for family leaders.

This outcome represented at least a partial win for everyone: staff who found work at the vendor agency took similar positions with improved pay, while case-management customers benefited from the experience and personal connections those staff brought. The state, for its part, was able to move into a more strategic role, having freed up resources for organization- and community-level networking and health assurance.

Engaging with Core Values
Organizational change draws energy from well-articulated shared values. One way to articulate the values is to ask multiple internal

and external stakeholder groups (leadership, staff, specific community partners and community members) at the start of a large change process, in multiple ways, what matters to them. When these groups gain clarity about the organization's values and purpose at the beginning of a large change process, they will be motivated to contribute to the change.

The local health department in Volusia County, Florida, provides an equity-based example. The Volusia County Health Department used an in-depth assessment for all staff to provide insights into what training and supports would be needed to centralize best practices in equity throughout the organization. Simultaneously, leadership went on an extensive visiting tour across the community to better understand the most pressing issues facing residents. Taken together, these streams of work made values clearer and engaged staff in the challenging first steps toward organizational change.

When you find common threads of purpose that excite and motivate, you begin to create a revised group identity. These values will be the quiet, certain center as systems and ways of thinking change. What makes transformational organizational change stick is a commitment to active learning, with dedicated time and space to reimagine, challenge, disagree, test, reflect, and reiterate the design. When an organization attempts large-scale change around a vision without first digging deep into common values, there can be an identity conflict at later stages of implementation, and a disconnect between how the change effort is being operationalized and how it sounded at the start.

Describing the Future State

It is important that throughout the change process, agreed-upon values of the organization stay the same. Change is about reimagining outcomes, but not often about core purpose and the things that matter most to an agency or a community. Part of the change effort should be to ask what is possible and spend time imagining collective hopes and dreams, especially those of the communities in which the agency or organization is engaged. Your efforts will benefit from both big, audacious visions—that stakeholders, leaders, and staff can get excited about—and more tangible, practical statements of future impacts and outcomes, what Heath and Heath call "destination postcards" in their book *Switch: How to Change Things When Change Is Hard*.[2]

An organizational vision should be compelling, clear, urgent (without provoking unhelpful anxiety), and values-driven. The values and vision should be in regular circulation with stakeholders to stay fresh and engaging.

The health department in Black Hawk, Iowa, provides another example from our ELPH program. In Black Hawk, leaders set a goal of shifting their agency's direct service model to one that focused on more upstream efforts, driving equity across community systems. The department worked internally to build that capacity with the help of the ELPH National Program Office and equity consultants. This new functional capacity has helped the agency integrate a systems-thinking approach. Black Hawk Health Department, with cross-sector partners in education, housing, and human services, has been re-examining the design of programs and services to better center equity, and in particular racial equity. Leaders started with the vision of all community residents enjoying optimal health and human development. Then they grounded their "future state" image in the places where residents play, work, learn, and worship. Last, they articulated that their internal organization would engage with equity concepts in personal, meaningful ways to guide policy design, surveillance, and operational practices more effectively.

Exploring Strategies

Strategy is your plan for how to win, the approaches you will take to achieve the future state. Vision describes the destination, but strategy describes things you will do to find and travel the path. Many health departments that have strategic plans work on a long-term schedule. Steps in the process include conducting a community health assessment, formulating the strategic plan for the agency, and then repeating the process in three or four years. The private sector largely has switched to a continual strategy cycle.

In her article "Putting Leadership Back into Strategy,"[3] Cynthia Montgomery argues that strategy development should be a dynamic process with a goal to continually create value. Most of the examples in this chapter are from this type of process, built around a focused new role or value transformation, as opposed to a general, three-year agency-wide plan, perhaps undertaken to meet an external requirement.

Effective strategic planning means considering carefully who wants the results you have in view, and who has a stake in any plan to deliver those results. Whose engagement in strategy development will influence implementation later? Who needs some control over the process? Who has decision-making power? Who has the power to execute or block the new strategy? Who has a perspective that has been missed in the past?

Trust is a key input and is essential to "co-creation" of plans. And co-creation of plans in turn creates trust as an output, trust you will be relying on later when you need support for the decisions that follow. Developing good strategies requires truth-telling and listening. The most valuable, paradigm-shifting strategies are accessible only to teams that have learned to support and challenge each other through constructive conflict and complexity.

(Re)Consider Organizational Structure: Functional Capacity Needs and Teams

Organizational structures are human designs, put in place to execute strategies. The more transformational your change, the more likely it is that structure change will help. Leadership has a key role in aligning structures to support the people who execute the strategy.

Several things can complicate your change. You should expect a long period of adaptation as people hash out their concerns, open up to new possibilities, say goodbye to their comfortable, familiar work, and move into a learning mindset with a new team. Structure change should help clarify roles if you are patient. Bring new teams together intentionally in a way that generates growth. Know that productivity will go down before it goes up. Let the process unfold and look for other structural adaptations to emerge that align with the new strategies.

The Chatham County Public Health Department in North Carolina offers an illustration of the strategy–structure relationship. The agency has long provided direct clinical services, but the emergence of additional clinical options in the county has made this role less critical than it once was for the health department. The organization saw this as an opportunity to focus county-wide attention and resources on upstream factors. Among its new population health initiatives is a cohort-based longitudinal community assessment that follows a representative sample of Chatham households over time to assess changes in health and socioeconomic status. In 2020, the community cohort was used to provide decision makers with real-time information about the early impacts of COVID-19, including positivity rates, adherence to public health guidance, access to care, and changes in economic and employment status.

New functional teams have two significant scopes of work related to the change process. First, they should be engaged in intentional individual and team development, allowing plenty of time and support for change efforts. Second, team members should co-create the role and broad scope of work for the functional team with (internal and external) stakeholders. Many of our state and local partners have found that their existing connections to external community groups in particular are insufficient, and that new teams have a key role in further developing those relationships.

Cultivating Change Agents to Guide the Change Process

Through the early stages of understanding and planning for organizational change, some staff members will demonstrate a high degree of readiness for coming changes by taking on leadership functions of various kinds: cheerleading, vision articulation, problem-solving, ideating. These employees are potential change agents, and you should cultivate them. They can help guide others through the planning and implementation stages. Help them learn how to use team-building strategies and facilitation skills to determine the scope of work for the newly established functional teams in ways that align with the new organizational strategies. Change agents can serve as ambassadors for change and can help deliver communications from and to leadership, across teams and divisions, and even to community partners.

Organizational Change through Team Trust

Successful teams have a high degree of trust among members that fuels their collective ability to manage large-scale change efforts and achieve great impacts. In *Smart Leaders, Smarter Teams*, Roger Schwartz argues that leaders and teams need to change the way they think, not just what they do. In his mutual learning mindset, teams overcome differences by bridging, not compromising. Bridging differences requires team members to understand more deeply and pay attention to where assumptions differ so that pathways for aligning interests emerge. Conflict is understood as what happens when different people advocate for different solutions from diverse perspectives. Rather than taking sides or activating turf wars, teams get clear, tell the truth, stay transparent, and stay in problem-solving mode. When conflict is viewed as natural and healthy rather than dysfunctional or negative, the conditions are established for authentic dialogue and learning. Differences become opportunities for learning, while learning fosters trust and expands team capacity to guide transformational change.

During the COVID-19 pandemic, outbreaks occurred across colleges and universities and in-person learning was abandoned in many locations. In environments where trust was low, campus administrations often worked independently and became misaligned with their communities, with predictable results. In our Champaign-Urbana, Illinois, team's experience, because of high levels of established trust, the local university worked in partnership with the health department on a comprehensive and rigorous COVID-19 testing strategy that quickly became a national model.

In organizational change efforts, it is preferable to task functional teams with sorting through current state programs, services, outreach, and other areas of work, then cross-walking them with new strategies and ultimately making recommendations to leadership about how this could translate to a future state that reflects the new vision and strategies. Design trust-building into the development and launch of those teams, and you will harness critical trust built through the co-creation approach.

Team-Building

Several variables can influence how much time and effort should be dedicated to team-building activities (including size of the team, where team members work, and whether team members have previously worked together), but you certainly should invest time in the process. Team members have individual needs, desires, and motivations, and adjustment periods vary from person to person. Allow ample time and space to talk through personal feelings related to change. Normalize that change preferences are different and that change is experienced differently by different people.

We all wear figurative masks to enable tasks to move smoothly, but transformation relies on trust and authenticity. You need enhanced working relationships that hook every individual into the commitment, because group candor and group problem-solving ability are at a premium in a transformational change process. Learning teams are different from purely task teams: learning teams have to know how to access and use each other's viewpoints, skills, and perspectives in order to fuel team knowledge acquisition and problem-solving.

Team Culture

Team culture is not something you can deliver by yourself as a leader, but you are responsible for it. Culture grows in the soil you till and responds to your care and pruning (or lack thereof). If the organizational change includes strategies related to organizational culture, then the changes need to be integrated into the structures of the organization (such as how information is shared, what is recognized and celebrated, or how meetings are organized and facilitated). In our maternal and child health work with the state of Tennessee, for example, the lead implementation team modeled how to use process evaluation efforts as opportunities to learn and grow. That modeling in turn positively affected how regional and local implementation teams approached partnering with community organizations. To create a culture of learning, leadership needs to attend to the team climate, modeling and highlighting constructive ways to share feedback, express concerns, and disagree.

Summary

Transformational change is humbling in its complexity, and a humble approach is indicated in guiding the process. Be bold in your vision, be bold in your decision-making, aim high for big new opportunities, but be humble and patient in your implementation. Expect to fail often, prepare to learn from those failures, then adjust and iterate patiently. The journey from near-extinction to prized community asset in Lubbock, Texas, was not a straight line for the public health agency. It zigged and zagged, collecting partners and building on small victories and maximizing unforeseen opportunities. To discern your desired role, and to know your strategy, takes a special kind of vision that discerns opportunity in what otherwise might look like confusion or disaster.

Systems change requires leaders who can guide collective value-setting and visioning, and then inspire others to join the effort. It takes an ability to switch seamlessly between the big-picture strategic view and the operational tasks that make change happen, all while paying close attention to the human qualities that either support or sabotage well-intentioned change efforts. Continuous communication about why the change effort is important and aligning the rationale with what is meaningful to various stakeholders are vital for change efforts to succeed.

In public health, it is important to master leadership skills in change management, no matter your authority status. The persistent, complex challenges that the field faces require passion and an adaptive skill set to disrupt the status quo and dismantle systems that span multiple sectors that no longer serve their purpose, all while motivating and working skillfully through others to achieve collective goals. In building our collective capacity to lead change effectively, we are stepping forward as a field to assert our value: ensuring that all members of our communities can thrive and experience health and well-being.

References

1. Crystal Conde, "Keeping Lubbock Healthy," *Texas Medicine* 108, no. 1 (2012): 39–43, https://www.texmed.org/Template.aspx?id=23294.
2. Chip Heath and Dan Heath, *Switch: How to Change Things When Change Is Hard.* (Crown Business, 2010).
3. Cynthia A. Montgomery, "Putting Leadership Back into Strategy," *Harvard Business Review* 86, no. 1 (2008): 54–60, https://hbr.org/2008/01/putting-leadership-back-into-strategy.

6

STRATEGIC SKILLS IN FOCUS:
▶ *Justice, Equity, Diversity, and Inclusion*

Leading with a Health Equity Lens

JEWEL MULLEN

PUBLIC LEADERSHIP FOR HEALTH EQUITY should be thought of as advancing what society does collectively for all people to be healthy. Adding that one word, *all*, to the 1988 Institute of Medicine (IOM) definition of public health concisely frames equity as the essence of our profession.[1] Traditional capabilities of governmental public health leadership, such as laboratory sciences, administration, surveillance, and performance management, are core technical functions. However, they are insufficient for achieving equity. The addition of the seemingly simple word *all* to the IOM definition also calls for leadership that is visionary, strategic, and transformative. That is because ensuring that all people can be as healthy as possible is a principle of social justice. It requires leaders to employ deliberative, value-based decision-making that is informed by sociopolitical history and the understanding of the roots of structural inequality, in order to serve individual and community well-being. In doing so, leaders may confront challenges to their personal ethics— their beliefs about merit, personal responsibility, the role of government, and justice. Those are complex considerations for which there is not a simple playbook.

Jewel Mullen, *Leading with a Health Equity Lens* In: *Building Strategic Skills for Better Health: A Primer for Public Health Professionals*. Edited by: Michael R. Fraser and Brian C. Castrucci, Oxford University Press.
© de Beaumont Foundation 2024. DOI: 10.1093/oso/9780197744604.003.0007

Nearly half a century ago, epidemiologist Dan Beauchamp suggested that public health is a way of doing justice, not merely a technical activity.[2] In promoting the idea that a justice approach is an ethical paradigm, he also recognized that the multiple factors that affect health are wide-ranging social problems. Beauchamp's framing was echoed by Harvard professor Nancy Krieger, who described social justice as a foundation of public health;[3] by Braveman, who called equity an ethical principal tied to human rights;[4] and by the World Health Organization Task Group on Equity, Equality and Human Rights, which stated in its report that the capability of every person to be healthy is central to social justice.[5]

Each of those assertions of the link between public health and justice also is reflected in Healthy People 2020, which reminded the nation that health equity, "the attainment of the highest level of health for all people," demands that we value everyone equally and act deliberately about eliminating past and ongoing injustices.[6] Those injustices, the initiative posits, are responsible for structural inequities, "the personal, interpersonal, institutional, and systemic drivers—such as, racism, sexism, classism, able-ism, xenophobia, and homophobia—that make those identities salient to the fair distribution of health opportunities and outcomes."[6]

Despite this long-standing view that public health is social justice, the will and capability to advance health equity, even among leaders who consider themselves committed to it, are not necessarily instinctive. Personal and organizational factors can get in the way or create gaps in understanding. One example of a personal factor is the mental trap that allows people to reinforce their positive self-image with thoughts like, "The proof that I believe in equity is that I believe everyone should be treated equally—and I always strive to do so." Leaders must understand the difference between equality and equity, be able to explain it, and then foster equitable systems and approaches that include undoing discriminatory policies and practices. They must discern that the equivalent allocation of resources to people without consideration of what they require for optimal health (equality) is not the same as apportionment that affords opportunities for all recipients to benefit fully from them (equity).

Disparities in access have resulted, for example, as municipalities established systems for all people to access COVID-19 testing or treatment without proactively planning for people and communities who lacked information about, transportation to, and the ability to register for, services.[7,8] Treating people equitably may require distributing more of a resource to those who lack it or have been prevented from acquiring it than to those who have traditionally benefitted from having more. It also calls for removal of barriers that keep people and groups from achieving their best possible outcomes. The associated goal is to narrow the avoidable health gap between those with the greatest abundance and power and those with the greatest need.

A second personal factor required for leading with an equity lens is empathy, the ability to see and understand others' thoughts and feelings. As a cognitive competency that can be learned, empathy is a professional state that requires self-awareness and facilitates human exchange.[9] Leaders who lack empathy may harbor blind spots that prevent them from embracing public health as a social value. Such leaders may place blame and accountability for social or structural disadvantage on those experiencing it. Empathy helps cultivate insight that a person's (or community's) vulnerabilities likely resulted from unjust laws, policies, and practices, and not individual failings. By upending the notion that people and groups can succeed if they just work harder, follow rules, or adopt healthier behaviors, empathy and insight should foster a leader's commitment to addressing people's needs. Yaseen suggests that "bias, race-, sex-, and class-ism, as well as stigma, all work as barriers to empathy" or can stifle leaders' engagement with people for whose well-being they are responsible.[9]

Another personal factor that leaders must cultivate is commitment to public accountability. Public accountability orients a leader to taking actions to undo injustice. Accountable leaders embrace promoting and restoring justice. They avoid an "I didn't break them, so I am not responsible for fixing them" attitude about people and communities. By highlighting growing evidence of the economic costs associated with health disparities, they promote advancing equity as a demonstration of accountability to all of society.[10,11]

Public health leaders must nurture their individual commitment, capability, and accountability to advance equity and to ensure that their agencies are effectively doing so. That is because personal factors may also manifest at an organizational level. For example, misconstruing equality as equity may occur across a public health agency. Such groupthink engenders agency policies and practices centered on equality rather than a justice-informed approach to public health. When that happens, or when empathy is absent from an organization's culture, an agency will be ill suited to promote health equity.

Organizational empathy aids development of policies and practices that are responsive to people and groups representing different races and ethnicities, as well as people with dissimilar languages, beliefs, values, and practices. Those differences are reflections of diversity. The ability to accommodate languages, values, and practices across diverse groups reflects cultural competence. Making cultural competence an agency priority may protect against equality-focused public health practice that might be unfair or ineffective for groups of people and communities.

Leadership for health equity must be grounded in fairness, empathy, and cultural competence, and none of those practices emerges through technical approaches alone. As with technical skills, these practices may seem somewhat methodological. However, approaches to them cannot be standardized. Leaders must have insight into, and confront, their own values, beliefs, biases, and knowledge gaps. Leading with a health equity lens requires sidelining personal ideologies and accepting that one does not have all the answers. It also requires promoting the imperative to undo injustices that are rooted in historic and, in some circumstances, ongoing social and structural inequities. Leadership for health equity, such as that required to address poverty, drug misuse, racism, poor education, and environmental hazards, is therefore an adaptive challenge.

As described by Heifetz, such challenges have no simple or proven solutions, identified expertise, clear leader, or single responsible authority.[12] Tackling inequity is a challenge that occurs in a context— usually more than one context at a time—requiring that leaders develop capacity to traverse a social-ecological framework for health.

It places people and communities, rather than leaders and their agencies, at the center. It opens the possibility for solutions to come from within communities. It interrogates beliefs, disrupts power structures, and reorients the hierarchy in relationships and roles. It calls for work that crosses disciplines. It takes time. It threatens to erode the walls and foundations that preserve silos in organizations and in social and political domains; those siloed systems are the status quo that might contain inequitable policy and practice. Leaders who break down the silos must replace them with something more effective. While there is no simple playbook for such transformation, a strategic public health skill set provides a way forward for thinking about which structures promote change and the outcomes those transformations can achieve.

The nine strategic skills represent the competencies that guide leading with a health equity lens. As a composite, they provide a framework for tackling the adaptive challenges associated with addressing social and structural determinants of health, and they inform leadership decisions. Each is necessary, none alone is sufficient, and they are interdependent. Systems thinking and change management are the bedrocks. Whether focused on work inside an agency or externally, those two skills guide a leader's approach to complexity. Complexity is inherent to managing change across numerous stakeholders in the context of their multiple shared or conflicting relationships, beliefs, histories, practices, and desired outcomes.

Applying the strategic skills, a public health leader can use insights about those intricacies to aid decisions on the selection, sequencing, timing, and pace of an initiative. Those insights may help uncover the potential for poorly planned and implemented evidence-based public health policy to increase rather than mitigate disparities or inequities, to erode partnerships rather than solidify them. As an example, although state primary seatbelt laws have been shown to narrow racial differences in seatbelt use, such legislation has led to a disproportionately higher rate of legal citations among Blacks than among Whites. Engaging stakeholders from minoritized communities alongside law enforcement when developing these laws can inform an approach that mitigates discriminatory policing and the possible social, emotional, and physical harm that might follow.[13,14]

Given that there can be multiple perspectives on how to advance equity, leaders must be able to communicate effectively to organize stakeholders around a shared vision for achieving it. Engaging the community in problem-solving and policy engagement, and ensuring that all perspectives are incorporated, is fundamental to upholding justice, equity, diversity, and inclusion (JEDI). In addition to helping craft persuasive messages, data-driven decision-making is essential for determining which health needs to prioritize, and for which populations. Data also help identify which strategic actions partners across multiple sectors might adopt, as well as the economic impacts of their doing so. None of this can be accomplished or sustained without sound resource management. While resource management may sound like a technical function, when it relates to leading with an equity lens, it is also strategic. Leaders might be responsible for communicating a vision for health equity and coordinating the associated work. However, they will not succeed as sole actors. Success starts with building an equity culture inside their agencies and ensuring that staff up and down and throughout their organizations also benefit from strategic skill development so that they can lead with formal and informal authority. Leaders must pave the way for their workforce to grow and become the partners, followers, and other visionaries who will help achieve an equity mission.

The Centers for Disease Control and Prevention's *Practitioner's Guide for Advancing Health Equity* lists the following seven questions that public health officials and their organizations can ask to inform their equity-related capacity and decision-making.[15] As indicated in italics, each question links to at least one strategic skill.

1. Where are we now? *Systems and strategic thinking, data-driven decision-making*
2. How can we institutionalize our organizational commitment to advance health equity? *Change management, resource management*
3. How can funding decisions advance our health equity efforts? *Data-driven decision-making, policy engagement, JEDI*

4. How can we build a skilled and diverse workforce committed to health equity? *JEDI, resource management*
5. How can we integrate health equity into our products and service offerings? *Change management, policy engagement*
6. How can our partnerships and community outreach efforts help to advance health equity? *Systems and strategic thinking, effective communication, policy engagement, JEDI*
7. What are our next steps? *All nine strategic skills*

Even when armed with framing questions for capacity to advance equity efforts, the leader's dilemma may be determining how to get started. The answer is to start with oneself, one's own learning and commitment, to lead others. The Institute for Healthcare Improvement describes leading for health equity as "a personal journey that needs to be undertaken as a group."[16] The importance of authentic, insightful organizational leadership cannot be underestimated. Staff need to experience leadership commitment as demonstrable support from the authority that helps them undertake the adaptive challenge of advancing equity.

What does that commitment look like? It is a leader's declaration that equity is a strategic priority for the organization. It can include incorporating equity and related principles into an organization's vision, mission, strategy, and culture. It means ordering the steps to advance equity, not getting stuck in trying to redefine it, because experts already have defined health equity many times over. It is reflected in a leader's transparency about her own path to learning about social determinants of health and their roots in social and structural inequality, including racism. Commitment also includes establishing internal policies and procedures to recruit and sustain a diverse workforce and promote their professional well-being. It emerges through adoption, even if incremental, of standards for culturally and linguistically appropriate services (CLAS). It means being deliberate about understanding the origins of disparities and inequities among the people and communities one's organization is accountable to, which requires collection of data (on processes and outcomes) by race, ethnicity, and language. It must be accompanied by building partnerships with communities, responding to their feedback, and learning how to engage effectively with them. It demands institutionalizing those actions in consistent organizational practice and policy. Incorporating all those steps into an effective state or community health improvement process puts equity, people, and communities at the center of a leader's work and creates a framework for measuring outcomes related to health, economics, and policy development.

Leading public health with a health equity lens may seem like a daunting task. It does not have to be. It is fundamentally leadership on behalf of all people, communities, and society. Public health's mission is to ensure that people can be healthy. The imperative for equity calls for acting so that all people have that opportunity. All of society benefits when that happens.

Like responses to natural disasters, pandemics, environmental catastrophes, or a rising obesity epidemic, applying an equity lens entails leadership in the face of risk, uncertainty about outcomes, resource constraints, competing priorities, and political pressures. It forces embracing the possibility of failure while hoping for the celebration of successfully promoting people's health and safety. That is a duality which is complex, risky, rewarding—and often fun. A strategic skill set helps leaders navigate that combination to advance health equity while building a thriving workforce and engaging with partners to get the work done. Fun? Perhaps it helps to think of leading with an equity lens as a dance. As public leadership expert Dean Williams suggests, "Real leadership is fundamentally an interactive art in which the leader is dancing with the context, the problem, the factions, and the objectives."[17] In this case, the objective is optimal health for all.

References

1. Institute of Medicine, Committee for the Study of the Future of Public Health, *The Future of Public Health* (Washington, DC: National Academies Press, 1988).
2. Dan E. Beauchamp, "Public Health as Social Justice," *Inquiry* 13, no. 1 (1976): 3–14, www.jstor.org/stable/29770972.
3. Nancy Krieger and Anne-Emanuelle Birn, "A Vision of Social Justice as the Foundation of Public Health: Commemorating 150 Years of the

Spirit of 1848," *American Journal of Public Health* 88, no. 11 (1998): 1603–1606, https://pubmed.ncbi.nlm.nih.gov/9807523/.

4. Paula A. Braveman et al., "Health Disparities and Health Equity: The Issue Is Justice," *American Journal of Public Health* 101, suppl. 1 (2011): S149–S155, https://www.ncbi.nlm.nih.gov/pmc/articles/PMC3222512/.

5. Karien Stonks et al., *Social Justice and Human Rights as a Framework for Addressing Social Determinants of Health: Final Report of the Task Group on Equity, Equality, and Human Rights* (Copenhagen: World Health Organization, 2016), http://www.euro.who.int/__data/assets/pdf_f ile/0006/334356/HR-task-report.pdf.

6. "Disparities," HealthyPeople.gov, Office of Disease Prevention and Health Promotion, https://www.healthypeople.gov/2020/about/foundat ion-health-measures/Disparities.

7. Lily Rubin-Miller et al., "COVID-19 Racial Disparities in Testing, Infection, Hospitalization, and Death: Analysis of Epic Patient Data," Kaiser Family Foundation, https://www.kff.org/coronavirus-covid-19/ issue-brief/covid-19-racial-disparities-testing-infection-hospitalization-death-analysis-epic-patient-data/.

8. Consuelo H. Wilkins et al., "A Systems Approach to Addressing COVID-19 Health Inequities," *NEJM Catalyst* 2, no. 1 (2021), https://catalyst. nejm.org/doi/pdf/10.1056/CAT.20.0374.

9. Adrianna E. Foster and Zimri S. Yaseen, *Teaching Empathy in Healthcare: Building a New Core Competency* (New York: Springer International Publishing, 2019), https://doi.org/10.1007/978-3-030-29876-0.

10. James N. Weinstein et al., *Communities in Action: Pathways to Health Equity* (Washington, DC: National Academies of Sciences, Engineering, and Medicine, 2017), http://www.nap.edu/.

11. Ani Turner, *The Business Case for Racial Equity: A Strategy for Growth* (W. K. Kellogg Foundation and Altarum, 2018), http://www.businesscaseforr acialequity.org.

12. Ronald A. Heifetz, *Leadership without Easy Answers* (Cambridge, MA: Belknap Press, 1998).

13. Nathaniel C. Briggs et al., "Seat Belt Law Enforcement and Racial Disparities in Seat Belt Use," *American Journal of Preventive Medicine* 31, no. 2 (2006): 135–141, https://pubmed.ncbi.nlm.nih.gov/16829330/.

14. ACLU and ACLU of Florida, *Racial Disparities in Florida Safety Belt Law Enforcement*, January 2016, https://www.aclu.org/sites/default/files/fie ld_document/racial_disparities_in_florida_safety_belt_law_enforce ment_final_02012016.pdf.

15. Centers for Disease Control and Prevention, Division of Community Health, "Building Organizational Capacity to Advance Health Equity," in *A Practitioner's Guide for Advancing Health Equity: Community Strategies*

for Preventing Chronic Disease (Atlanta, GA: US Department of Health and Human Services, 2013), 6–9, https://www.cdc.gov/nccdphp/dnpao/state-local-programs/health-equity-guide/pdf/health-equity-guide/Health-Equity-Guide-sect-1-1.pdf.

16. Institute for Healthcare Improvement, "Improving Healthcare Equity: 5 Guiding Principles for Health Care Leaders," March 1, 2018, http://www.ihi.org/communities/blogs/improving-health-equity-5-guiding-principles-for-health-care-leaders.

17. Dean Williams, *Real Leadership: Helping People and Organizations Face Their Toughest Challenges* (San Francisco, CA: Berrett-Koehler, 2005).

Effective Communication

RENATA SCHIAVO AND MAYELA ARANA

The Role of Communication in Public Health: An Introduction

Communication is part of everyday life and therefore is an essential component of the work of public health practitioners. With its emphasis on building bridges, bolstering confidence and leadership skills, and engaging individuals, communities, policymakers, and other stakeholders, communication is key to fostering behavioral, social, organizational, and policy change at different levels of society.[1] Ultimately, effective communication contributes to improving population and community health outcomes, building social support for healthy behaviors, engaging vulnerable and marginalized populations, advancing health equity, addressing misinformation, and promoting or sustaining healthy behaviors and related social norms and policies.

Yet only communication interventions and approaches that are grounded in systematic planning frameworks, sound principles, theories, and strategies are likely to achieve short- and long-term results.[1-3] While many skills useful in improvisation can be helpful in communication—such as the ability to listen to, and assume the

Renata Schiavo and Mayela Arana, *Effective Communication* In: *Building Strategic Skills for Better Health: A Primer for Public Health Professionals*. Edited by: Michael R. Fraser and Brian C. Castrucci, Oxford University Press.
© de Beaumont Foundation 2024. DOI: 10.1093/oso/9780197744604.003.0008

best in, others; to show empathy; and to connect emotionally and intellectually[4]—there should be no improvisation in the practice of communication. Increasingly, communication planning is an essential skill for public health practitioners, which, among others, points to the role communication plays in (1) engaging and building trust among communities and different publics, and (2) facilitating processes and interventions across the many professions and disciplines that contribute to the public health field.[1]

For example, during the COVID-19 pandemic in New York State, local health departments were required to employ a variety of strategies to communicate COVID-related information. Public health professionals had to practice humility through moments of uncertainty in the face of constantly changing guidelines and executive orders. In addition to the governor's daily briefings, local health departments in the state set up online community dashboards to inform community members about new mandates and precautions. Some created hotlines for the public and others participated in briefings set up by county leadership. These communication efforts among community-based organizations, governmental agencies, and the public were essential in making possible the work of local departments of health to set up widespread testing, effectively trace positive cases, provide wraparound services, and ultimately flatten the COVID-19 curve in New York during the summer of 2020.[6]

Another example suggests that, during the Ebola epidemic in 2014–2015, a participatory communication planning process was instrumental in building bridges with local communities by engaging residents to design solutions and communicate information.[6] This ultimately helped "governments in low-trust settings overcome their credibility deficit when promoting public welfare."[7] This type of intervention resulted in "increasing adherence to safety precautions, support for contentious control policies, and general trust in government."[7] It also pointed to the link between effective communication and the perceived or actual credibility of those who are engaged in the communication design, implementation, and evaluation process, who in this case also included residents.[6,7]

The good news is that there is no shortage of planning frameworks[1,6,8,9] for social and behavioral change that integrate theories and models for effective communication and multilevel interventions, participatory processes, and the role of persuasion, among others.[10,11] While these frameworks can differ in some of their steps and cycles, at the core of well-designed and implemented communication interventions and approaches are a number of common and shared principles,[1] including (1) recognizing the need to be inclusive of vulnerable and marginalized populations; (2) understanding that communication planning is a strategic process that goes beyond messages and materials, and should include group-specific goals, objectives, and strategies, as well as be engaging to key stakeholders; and (3) acknowledging that the system-driven nature of communication interventions calls for addressing barriers and behaviors at different levels of society, ultimately making healthy behaviors the easy behaviors. These principles resonate with recent public health agendas both in the United States and internationally[12] and inform the many ways communication can help address health and social issues.

In the age of disinformation, one of the most important ways that communication can help is by "building social support networks"[12] both in communities and online. Social media has become a persistent and crucial part of society. With this trend, and in the absence of adequate interventions, misinformation may become an uncontrollable problem leading to people-made crises like vaccine hesitancy and its increased inequities.

Consider the case of Barbara, a young mother of a one-month-old baby girl, who is struggling with the decision to immunize her child. She hears conflicting information on the safety and benefits of vaccines and is unsure about what and whom to believe: her local health department, her physician, other mothers in her community, her family members, and/or the information she reads and shares on social media.[1]

While communication can provide an element of social support to inform Barbara about making the right decision to immunize her child,[1] it will only work if the communication relies on getting to know Barbara and listening to and engaging her, her peers, and the many people or media from which she seeks information and reassurance on this topic.[1] For example, what is Barbara's lifestyle? What do mothers in her peer group think about immunization? Is access to vaccines a perceived barrier? What kind of support does she get from her family on important decisions? What does she read? What media does she use? Who does she listen to? Does she have a good relationship with her daughter's clinicians?

The list of questions goes on and on, suggesting the need to design a comprehensive communication intervention that, for example, includes (1) advocating for new policies to control misinformation on health issues, (2) strengthening interpersonal communication skills of clinicians, (3) improving the quality and accuracy of media coverage through tailored outreach to national and local media, (4) removing systemic barriers to immunization and/or vaccine access within Barbara's community, (5) fostering community engagement to give voice to local champions (e.g., parents who immunize their children, women's groups in support of immunization) both online and in community settings, and (5) "engaging hesitant parents and vaccine refuters."[1,13]

Increasingly in the twenty-first century, being motivated to adopt and maintain any kind of behavior is linked to the actual or perceived intimacy of relationships,[14] which in turn can influence the ability to engage others and affect beliefs, attitudes, and behaviors both online and offline. Key to effective communication is to create the feeling that "I heard it everywhere,"[1] so that public health practitioners can reassure mothers like Barbara, support their decision-making, and occupy the media and community spaces that can otherwise become filled with misinformation.

For example, during the COVID-19 pandemic, public health professionals were tasked with addressing conflicting information and disinformation, contributing to the ongoing *infodemic*, a term that describes the overabundance of information that may emerge during an epidemic[15] or in relation to other health issues, such as the safety and effectiveness of vaccines. This overabundance of information can make it difficult to distinguish facts from fiction and can "lead to confusion and ultimately mistrust in governments and the public health response."[16] This was evident during the COVID-19 pandemic on topics ranging from willingness to comply (or lack thereof) with mask and social distancing measures, hesitancy to be vaccinated against the virus, and adherence with routine preventative health activities.[13,17,18]

This chapter focuses on effective communication as a core strategic skill for public health, which often intersects with, and in many cases is foundational to, the other areas in the strategic skills for public health framework. It examines key features of effective communication within the context of behavioral and social change communication, and the role of storytelling in communication. Finally, it provides practical recommendations for implementation and leadership.

What Is Effective Communication?

Effective communication is an "interactive process of partnership and dialogue" to exchange information, ideas, and methods with a variety of groups to create suitable communication strategies and interventions to influence behaviors, policies, and social norms.[19] It centers the values, environments, and priorities of specific groups in engaging with different levels of society to address health and social issues and to contribute to removing barriers to healthy behaviors. It may utilize a wide array of formats to better reach groups of interest.

"Effective communication is participatory in its nature and seeks to empower intended groups and communities to create long-lasting and transformative change."[19] This can range from communicating about policy options with legislators, to engaging with communities to bring about grassroots social change around civic issues, to discussing health information in counseling and clinical settings.

Regardless of the communication setting, many of the principles of effective communication resonate with key aspects of interpersonal communication, which not only involves the exchange of information among key participants, but also requires an in-depth understanding of the priorities, values, skills, social factors, policies, barriers, and opportunities that may influence behavior change. Regardless of specific media, an attempt should always be made to convey a feeling of mutual understanding and caring with all kinds of communication efforts, activities, and media.[1]

There are various key factors to consider when engaging in developing communication interventions. Understanding specific knowledge, attitudes, and beliefs on any given health or social issue of a group being sought to engage is an essential first step to developing personally relevant and community-driven communication. Working with communities and their leaders and effectively engaging them in the design, implementation, and evaluation of all interventions are also key to securing community awareness of health and social issues; improving community buy-in and compliance with recommended health behaviors; addressing issues of trust, cultural relevance and information transparency; and managing misinformation, among others.

In pandemics, epidemics, and emerging disease settings, community-based risk communication has long been a participatory approach that "includes two-way interaction with the community at every step of the risk mitigation process, right from the point of determining what issues should be addressed, and why."[20] Community mobilization and citizen engagement not only contribute to the adoption and sustainability of disease mitigation measures but also have "been credited as a strategy for providing additional community and public services during epidemics and disease outbreaks."[20] Most important, both in community and other communication settings, empathy (the ability to understand, share, and connect to someone's feelings and experiences by remembering moments in our lives in which we have felt the same way)[21] and cultural humility are key to creating bridges and making sure that communication is people-centered, displays a genuine respect for the values and preferences of the people being sought to engage, and ultimately helps advance equity in health and other human rights issues.

One key factor in effective communication is the process of reciprocation (a mutual exchange in which people acknowledge and respond to others' ideas and needs), which enhances feelings of trust, enables positive rapport, and facilitates positive interpersonal interaction.[22]

Research in the field of neuroscience explains that when engaging others in any kind of communication, the brain is implicitly and explicitly weighing consequences and benefits that may be relevant to making a value-based decision about behaviors.[23] Moreover, an increasing number of studies showcase that communication is bioactive [24,25] and as Siegel notes, communications can shape brain structure, influence immune function, and impact individual biology.[26]

This is why simply presenting facts is not enough to achieve behavioral change. In other words, how things are said is just as important as what is said.

Using theory-driven approaches can help increase the impact of a communication effort by increasing receptivity and building trust among intended groups. For example, the elaboration likelihood model (figure 7.1) posits that messages are processed through two distinct main pathways.[10,27] On one pathway, messages are perceived as deliberate, thoughtful, and more likely to produce enduring behavior change, while on the other pathway, messages rely on simple associations that lead to fast judgments that may result in less enduring changes in behavior.[10,27] Although some theoretical frameworks are more appropriate at different levels of the socioecological model with varying populations and cultures or may have resource and capacity

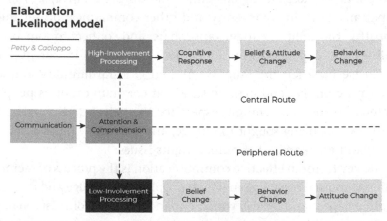

Figure 7.1. The elaboration likelihood model. Source: Wolswijk, Floris. "Elaboration Likelihood Model." July 21, 2014, https://floriswolswijk.com/elaboration-likelihood-model/. Redrawn with permission.

considerations, these approaches may help to organize one's thoughts and define the steps of wide-ranging communication efforts.

It is important to use a systematic approach to facilitate the understanding of social influences, including relationships with partners, family members, one's own community, and social norms and policies. This is key to effective communication and requires an iterative process of learning and adaptation.[28] At each level of the socioecological model (figure 7.2), there are influences that must be accounted for to communicate effectively and to adequately address health needs. These include a variety of social determinants of health as well as additional perceived or actual barriers to, and facilitators of, behavior change. Most important, because people at each level of the socioecological model of health also need to adopt and sustain behaviors, norms, and policies that are supportive of individual behavior change, communication interventions cannot be limited to the individual and interpersonal levels.

In fact, a key element in behavior change is social support. Perceived social support of a behavior is associated with behavioral adherence, which points to the importance of recognizing that differing social

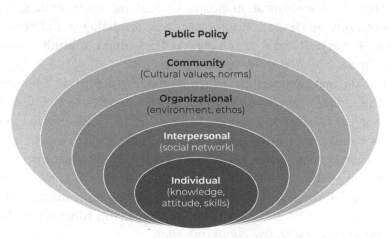

Figure 7.2. The socioecological model of health and influences on behavior change. Source: Coroiu, A., Moran, C., Campbell, T., Geller, A.C. (2020) Barriers and facilitators of adherence to social distancing recommendations during COVID-19 among a large international sample of adults. *PLOS One* 15(10): e0239795, Fig. 1, p. 6. https://doi.org/10.1371/journal.pone.0239795. License: CC BY 4.0.

networks may have contradictory knowledge, attitudes, and beliefs about behaviors,[27] and that these all need to be considered as part of a communication process. Creating supportive environments that stimulate learning and enable active participation not only leads to behavioral change, but also generates social movements and social change.[28]

In summary, effective communication is not simply about stating facts; it also requires establishing a connection that is meaningful and relevant to one's life. Taking these various aspects of effective communication into consideration facilitates the design of community-based interventions that resonate with, and engage, a variety of groups, ultimately leading to the implementation of new or existing policies, the creation of coalitions, the adoption and sustainability of new health behaviors, and other key results that can influence the health of the public and communities.

The Power of Stories

Telling stories is the best way to engage, teach, persuade, and even understand oneself and one's surroundings. Stories help reinforce positive cultural values and practices, actively involve others, and strengthen communication across professions, communities, and generations. Stories are an important tool for dialogue and engagement, behavioral and social change, and creating community ownership and social support for healthy behaviors.

Within the framework and forward-looking definition examined in this chapter for effective communication, stories can be used to engage, to catalyze analysis, to solve problems, and to build consensus rather than merely to convince. This approach ultimately challenges communities, coworkers, partners, family members, and others to analyze real-life issues and to discuss how to solve them.[29] This creates ownership, empowerment, and long-term sustainability of all solutions[20,30] and serves as a key leadership function and an essential trait of effective communication.

Leading with stories in interpersonal and group settings can create a safe space to share opinions, including potential dissent. For example, when the leader of a professional team tells a story, it may perpetuate past issues and problems or encourage creativity and innovation. One way to inspire the latter is to encourage team members, both in meetings and via email, to tell stories that illustrate how their work is helping further the organization's mission in addition to advancing overall public health outcomes. Similarly, telling a story about how a dissenting coworker changed minds on a past issue may also encourage participation and the flow of new ideas.[31]

Furthermore, because "showing instead of telling"[1] is an important mantra of effective communication, the power of a story can transcend interpersonal settings and can be used effectively across a variety of media and venues. For example, visual media and digital storytelling (media production facilitating the sharing of stories, such as web-based communication and audio and video podcasts) have steadily become an important component of public health interventions. Using relatable emotional content, a storyteller's point of view can be illustrated through effective visual media and digital interventions. As is true for all elements of effective communication, storytelling efforts should be designed to maximize community and stakeholder engagement. In addition, participatory media development, which engages communities, young people, and other key stakeholders in media design and content, is also likely to add trust and credibility to the information being discussed. This trend is currently happening via social media and in the dissemination of news through online interactions.[32]

As an example, in 2019, the New Mexico Department of Health launched a visual media and storytelling video series on opioid misuse. The department was seeking to remove stigma and to suggest "that we are all in this epidemic together." To connect people with community resources to help them deal with the epidemic,[33] the series tells the story of opioid misuse from three points of view—patients in treatment, those working with people in treatment, and those who have had loved ones affected by opioid misuse.

In another example, the National Association of County and City Health Officials collected stories about COVID-19 response efforts from local health departments in 2020. Once gathered and compiled, the stories illustrating the critical role of local health departments were shared with various stakeholder groups to generate national funding, to increase advocacy, and to raise the visibility of public health, especially at a time when public health officials were receiving backlash from the public.[34]

These examples, as well as many others, reinforce the importance of storytelling as an effective tool for public health practitioners while also exhibiting wide applications for a variety of health and social issues. Increased capacity-building and training on participatory planning, participatory media, storytelling, and media development may help address some of the challenges faced by public health professionals in the movement to institutionalize storytelling as an essential element of their public health communication approach and strategy.

Effective Communication Skills and Strategies for the Twenty-First Century

Increasingly, multisectoral partnerships are necessary to generate collective impact and improve local and public conditions. Collaborating with various stakeholders, forming coalitions, and engaging with communities and the public are needed to successfully roll out public health interventions and to take significant policy action. For example, in the early stages of the COVID-19 pandemic, many county health departments in New York leveraged existing relationships with local hospital systems, law enforcement, and community-based organizations to create testing centers, to enforce mask and social distancing ordinances, to provide support to local businesses, and to deliver wraparound services to community members who were required to quarantine.[5] Such relationships were essential to effectively communicate with a variety of groups daily to strengthen the health of the community and, in the case of COVID-19, to save lives.

Trusted relationships are key to effectively communicating evidence-based public health information, a process that has become increasingly challenging, especially with the rise in deliberate disinformation campaigns on the Internet and in other settings. Infodemic management is the process of communicating evidence-based interventions and making them understandable to the public.[15] This people-centered approach to combating the overwhelming problem of disinformation and mixed messaging seeks to increase self-efficacy and to provide skills used to identify misleading information, ultimately building communities that are less susceptible to potentially life-threatening information and behaviors. For example, media and virtual communication have been growing exponentially, but more Americans are wary of information received online.[35] Mass media and media advocacy can help bring even greater awareness to health issues and promote civic action.[28] While online communication, such as social media, can be suitable and even the preferred method of communication for various groups, communities must be empowered with necessary skills to identify and resist disinformation, and with the ability to amplify life-saving and accurate public health messaging in their social networks.[15]

State and local governmental public health agencies are often the drivers of change that affects the social, community-based, and economic determinants of health. Effective communication is an essential part of the interactive process that is required in public health leadership.[36] Only when practitioners work with multisectoral partners and engage community members can behavior change grow on a systemic level. Governmental public health workers must be able to engage in conversations about the well-being of vulnerable and marginalized populations in ways that are clear, credible, and thorough. Public health leadership should consider the use of tools like key group and stakeholder analysis, community dialogue, coalition-building, participatory planning, and other participatory methods to ensure that all perspectives are represented and to adequately tailor communication. Communicating effectively is a trait of a leader, not simply a tool for a leader to use. Effective communication is based on mutual trust, intimacy, and connection between individuals. Therefore, leaders must first listen to, and engage with, diverse groups to understand priorities and then design and generate a shared vision for health.[37]

As an organization begins planning ways to engage with communities, build coalitions, and influence policymakers, it must consider the following strategies to improve effective communication skills:

- Engage local communities and stakeholders in the communication design, implementation, and evaluation process to provide community members with true ownership of local solutions and to improve the cultural relevance and effectiveness of all communication.

- Use tools like key group and stakeholder analysis, community dialogue, and other participatory methods to understand the attitudes, beliefs, values, and priorities of the communities you seek to engage. Listen first, and then aim to establish or restore trust and long-term relationships, especially if working with vulnerable and marginalized communities that may have historical reasons for mistrust. Remember to analyze systemic barriers to behavioral change and other social factors, policies, and conditions that may prevent people from leading healthy and productive lives.

- Create communication interventions that engage key groups on achieving realistic and focused behavior change and remove social, environmental, and policy barriers to behavior adoption and sustainability.

- Focus on building social support around a behavior, because individuals are influenced by the support of others in their family, community, and workplace.

- Consider the appropriateness of the modality and setting of communication for different interventions and groups.

- Consider how possible the proposed behavior change may be for certain communities and individuals. For example, healthy nutrition is more difficult to achieve for people who don't have easy access to healthy and affordable food options, including the millions of Americans who live in food deserts. In this case, the community-based communication effort may be more effective if it is initially directed at influencing and engaging policymakers, companies, and other key stakeholders to make changes in the food environments of the communities.

- Strategically use mass media and virtual communications to influence policies, social norms, and health behaviors. Make sure that interventions and messages create the same feeling of relevance and connectedness that is key to effective interpersonal communication. Partner with local communities, patient groups, mothers' groups, and other organizations that represent everyday citizens to give voice to local champions who support healthy behaviors.

These are just a few examples of potential strategies for implementation. Ongoing work with communities and partners is likely to highlight many additional and/or completely different group- and community-specific ways to improve the effectiveness of communication and promote community ownership of local solutions, as well as the sustainability of behavioral and social results.

Summary

This chapter positions effective communication within the broader context of social and behavior change communication and provides practical recommendations and examples to implement effective communication skills while mitigating the effects of deliberate misinformation in the twenty-first century. Most importantly, this chapter examines the significance of empathy, storytelling, cultural humility, community and key group participation and engagement, equity, and other key factors influencing the dynamics of public health communication within the framework of the strategic skills for public health.

References

1. Renata Schiavo, *Health Communication: From Theory to Practice*, 2nd ed. (San Francisco, CA: Jossey-Bass, 2013).
2. Dolores Albarracín et al., "Persuasive Communications to Change Actions: An Analysis of Behavioral and Cognitive Impact in HIV Prevention," *Health Psychology* 22, no. 2 (2003): 166–177, https://www.ncbi.nlm.nih.gov/pmc/articles/PMC4803280/.
3. Timothy P. Gill and Sinead Boylan, "Public Health Messages: Why Are They Ineffective and What Can Be Done?" *Current Obesity Reports* 1 (2012): 50–58, https://link.springer.com/article/10.1007/s13 679-011-0003-6.

4. Jennifer Braunschweige, "Four Improv Techniques That Can Help You Communicate Better," *Fast Company*, November 21, 2016, https://www.fastcompany.com/3065230/four-improv-techniques-that-can-help-you-communicate-better.

5. Sarah Ravenhall et al., "New York State Local Health Department Preparedness for and Response to the COVID-19 Pandemic: An In-progress Review," *Journal of Public Health Management and Practice* 27, no. 3 (2021): 240–245, https://pubmed.ncbi.nlm.nih.gov/33570870/.

6. UNICEF, "Communication for Development," https://sites.unicef.org/cbsc/index_42328.html.

7. Lily L. Tsai LL, Benjamin S. Morse, and Robert A. Blair, "Building Credibility and Cooperation In Low-Trust Settings: Persuasion and Source Accountability in Liberia during the 2014–2015 Ebola Crisis," *Comparative Political Studies* 53 (2020): 1582–1618, https://journals.sage pub.com/doi/abs/10.1177/0010414019897698?journalCode=cpsa.

8. "Gateway to Health Communication," Centers for Disease Control and Disease Prevention, August 4, 2020, https://www.cdc.gov/healthco mmunication/index.html.

9. Everold Hosein, Will Parks, and Renata Schiavo, "Communication-for-Behavioral-Impact: An Integrated Model for Health and Social Change," in *Emerging Theories in Health Promotion Practice and Research: Strategies for Improving Public Health*, 2nd ed., eds. Ralph J. DiClemente, Richard A. Crosby, and Michelle C. Kegler (San Francisco, CA: Jossey-Bass, 2010).

10. Johns Hopkins University, "Social and Behavior Change Communication for Emergency Preparedness Implementation Kit," Health Communication Capacity Collaborative, 2021, https://healthc ommcapacity.org/hc3resources/social-behavior-change-communicat ion-emergency-preparedness-implementation-kit/.

11. Suruchi Sood et al., *Technical Guidance for Communication for Development Programmes Addressing Violence Against Children* (New York: UNICEF, 2019), https://www.unicef.org/media/73491/file/C4D-VAC-Technical-Guidance-2019.pdf.

12. Office of Disease Prevention and Health Promotion, U.S. Department of Health and Human Services, "Health Communication and Health Information Technology," in *Healthy People* 2020, https://www.health ypeople.gov/2020/topics-objectives/topic/health-communication-and-health-information-technology.

13. Renata Schiavo et al., "Grounding Evaluation Design in the Socio-ecological Model of Health; A Logic Framework for the Assessment of a National Routine Immunization Communication Initiative in Kyrgyzstan," *Global Health Promotion* 4, (2020): 1–10, https://pubmed.ncbi.nlm.nih.gov/32400250/.

14. Denise Solomon, Jennifer Theiss, *Interpersonal Communication: Putting Theory into Practice*, (New York, NY: Taylor & Francis, 2013).
15. World Health Organization, "Infodemic Management," 2020, https://www.who.int/teams/risk-communication/infodemic-management.
16. J. Hope Corbin et al. "A Health Promotion Approach to Emergency Management: Effective Community Engagement Strategies from Five Cases," *Health Promotion International* 36, suppl. 1 (2021): i24–i38, https://www.ncbi.nlm.nih.gov/pmc/articles/PMC8667549.
17. Rory Smith, Seb Cubbon, and Claire Wardle, "Under the Surface: Covid-19 Vaccine Narratives, Misinformation & Data Deficits on Social Media," *First Draft News*, November 12, 2020, https://firstdraftnews.org/long-form-article/under-the-surface-covid-19-vaccine-narratives-misinformation-and-data-deficits-on-social-media/.
18. Washington Post Editorial Board, "The Pandemic Is Triggering Another Disaster: Untreated Diseases," *Washington Post*, November 18, 2020, https://www.washingtonpost.com/opinions/global-opinions/the-pandemic-is-triggering-another-disaster-untreated-diseases/2020/11/18/d9d8dff0-2902-11eb-92b7-6ef17b3fe3b4_story.html?sf133963595=1.
19. de Beaumont Foundation, "Adapting and Aligning Public Health Strategic Skills," https://debeaumont.org/strategic-skills/.
20. Renata Schiavo, Karen M. Hilyard, and Ewart C. Skinner, "Community-Based Risk Communication in Epidemics and Emerging Disease Settings," in *Introduction to Global Health Promotion*, eds. R. S. Zimmerman, R. J. DiClemente, J. K. Andrus, E. Hosein, and Society of Public Health Education (SOPHE) (San Francisco, CA: Jossey-Bass, 2016), 272.
21. Helen Riess, *The Empathy Effect: Seven Neuroscience-Based Keys for Transforming the Way We Live, Love, Work, and Connect Across Differences* (Boulder, CO: Sounds True, 2018).
22. C. Warren, S. Becken, and A. Coghlan, "Using Persuasive Communication to Co-create Behavioural Change—Engaging with Guests to Save Resources at Tourist Accommodation Facilities," *Journal of Sustainable Tourism* 25, no. 7 (2016): 935–954, https://www.tandfonline.com/doi/abs/10.1080/09669582.2016.1247849?journalCode=rsus20.
23. Emily Falk and Christin Scholz, "Persuasion, Influence, and Value: Perspectives from Communication and Social Neuroscience," *Annual Review of Psychology* 69, no. 1 (2018): 329–356, https://www.annualreviews.org/doi/abs/10.1146/annurev-psych-122216-011821.
24. John Parrish-Sprowl, "Communication Systems under GAP," World Health Organization (online presentation, Global Health Communication Center, Indiana University), https://www.who.int/influenza_vaccines_plan/GAPIII_Session1_ParrishSprowl.pdf.

25. Louis Cozolino, *The Neuroscience of Human Relationships: Attachment and the Developing Social Brain*, 2nd ed. (New York: W.W. Norton, 2014).
26. Daniel J. Siegel, *The Developing Mind: How Relationships and the Brain Interact to Shape Who We Are*, 2nd ed. (New York: The Guilford Press, 2012).
27. Karen Glanz, Barbara K. Rimer, and K. Viswanath, *Health Behavior: Theory, Research, and Practice*, 5th ed. (New York: Jossey-Bass, 2015).
28. William Robert Avis, "Methods and Approaches to Understanding Behavior Change," *GSDRC Applied Knowledge Services* 1, no. 389 (2016): 1–25, http://gsdrc.org/wp-content/uploads/2016/08/HDQ1389.pdf.
29. Judi Aubel, *Stories-Without-An-Ending: An Adult Education Tool for Dialogue and Social Change* (The Grandmother Project and USAID, 2017), https://www.fsnnetwork.org/sites/default/files/stories_without_an_ending.pdf.
30. Renata Schiavo, "The Importance of Community-based Communication for Health and Social Change," *Journal of Communication in Healthcare: Strategies, Media, and Engagement in Global Health* 9, no. 1 (2016): 1–3, https://www.tandfonline.com/doi/full/10.1080/17538068.2016.1154755.
31. Harrison Monarth, "These Are Three Types of Stories That Leaders Need to Master," *Fast Company*, July 9, 2019, https://www.fastcompany.com/90373480/these-are-the-3-types-of-stories-that-leaders-need-to-master.
32. George Lăzăroiu, "The Social Construction of Participatory Media Technology," *Contemporary Readings in Law and Social Justice* 6, no 1. (2014): 104–109, https://heinonline.org/HOL/LandingPage?handle=hein.journals/conreadlsj6&div=13&id=&page=/.
33. "Real Life Stories: New Mexico Department of Health Launches New Video Series in Fight against Opioid Abuse," New Mexico Department of Health, July 9, 2019, https://nmhealth.org/news/information/2019/7/?view=776.
34. "Submit Your Stories about COVID-19 Response Efforts," National Association of County and City Health Officials (NACCHO), https://www.naccho.org/programs/our-covid-19-response/coronavirus.
35. Elisa Shearer and Elizabeth Grieco, "Americans Are Wary of the Role Social Media Sites Play in Delivering the News," Pew Research Center, October 2, 2019, https://www.journalism.org/2019/10/02/americans-are-wary-of-the-role-social-media-sites-play-in-delivering-the-news/.
36. Louis Rowitz, *Public Health Leadership: Putting Principles Into Practice* (Burlington, MA: Jones & Bartlett Learning, 2009).
37. Saskia Kelders et al., "Behavior Change Support Systems" (workshop proceedings, CEUR, Chicago, IL, June 3, 2015), http://ceur-ws.org/Vol-1369/.

8

Managing and Leading in a Public Health 3.0 Era

MICHAEL R. FRASER

DESPITE DISCUSSION AND DEBATE IN the literature on organizational behavior and management about whether leadership and management are two different concepts, a premise of this overview is that leadership and management simply reflect two different areas of focus for leaders. Traditionally, leadership is defined as the work of setting organizational direction, aligning resources to advance organizational strategy, and inspiring others to move an organization's strategy forward. Management is defined as the task-focused, operational, or administrative work in an organization. Table 8.1 summarizes some of the ways that the two concepts are differentiated in business literature.

These differences are important. Work with governmental public health agencies has shown that the current and future challenges facing governmental public health practice demand more leadership from public health practitioners and less management. While being a competent manager is important, too often the daily tasks of program administration and finance, personnel issues and supervision, and tactical budget and policy development consume most public

Michael R. Fraser, *Managing and Leading in a Public Health 3.0 Era* In: *Building Strategic Skills for Better Health: A Primer for Public Health Professionals*. Edited by: Michael R. Fraser and Brian C. Castrucci, Oxford University Press. © de Beaumont Foundation 2024. DOI: 10.1093/oso/9780197744604.003.0009

Table 8.1. Comparison of Areas of Emphasis for Leadership and Management

Leadership	Management
Strategy- and vision-focused[13]	Process- and present-focused[17]
Identifies needed changes, future-focused	Promotes the status quo
Sets direction, creates "shared vision"[14]	Follows the plan, develops the "how"[10]
"Doing the right thing"[10]	"Doing the thing right"[10]
Asks questions, identifies challenges[6]	Gives answers, solves problems
Broad in scope, cross-cutting/ horizontal[15]	Narrow in scope, vertical[15]
Creates value[16]	Counts value[16]
Creates circles of influence[16]	Creates circles of power[16]
Creates new systems, advances change[13]	Minimizes risk, keeps the current system operating[13]
Others are "human beings"[10]	Others are "human doings"[10]

health leaders with problem-solving tasks and administrative activities. An emphasis on management functions leaves less time to think strategically and diminishes the ability to position an agency to meet a complex and changing set of challenges. Governmental public health practice requires practitioners to be both effective leaders and effective managers. Rarely does the complexity and scope of public health practice require just "managing," and rarely does the volume and pace of public health work allow just "leading." These activities need to be integrated to move agencies forward in environments of constant change and as people face both persistent and emerging public health threats.

The first months of public health's response to COVID-19 provided a good example of the difference between leading and managing. Actions focused on "managing the response" instead of developing and supporting leadership to take on broad strategic issues and create a shared local-state-federal vision for measures that engaged and motivated others. The early focus on management included dealing with technical issues, such as supply chains and a shortage of personal protective equipment, determining how to get Americans off cruise ships abroad and then home, addressing mass-testing supply shortages, revising scientific guidance, distributing medications and other supplies, and procuring equipment. Lack of coordinated and clear national leadership left state and local officials on their own to acquire resources and to compete with other jurisdictions. Multiple local-to-federal pathways emerged for data reporting and solved immediate problems but did not strategically build on the need for data modernization and improved information technology infra-structure, an issue that state public health leaders have recognized for years. These tactical management issues consumed health officials' time but did little to instill confidence in the ability of these profes-sionals to prevent infection and end the pandemic. The only way to reach this kind of collective strategy is through effective leader-ship, and its absence led to profound and preventable consequences, including rising infection rates, significant illness, and death.

Public Health 3.0, a model used to describe contemporary govern-mental public health practice, builds on the past and spells out the need for the field to adapt and evolve.[8] Figure 8.1 depicts the evolution of public health practice that Public Health 3.0 represents, based on twentieth-century advances in public health and more recent develop-ments in the early twenty-first century. The challenge associated with the move to Public Health 3.0 should not be underestimated. Leading change and transformation efforts in government is difficult because the aim of a bureaucracy is to rationalize functions, to specialize tech-nical knowledge, and to routinize and standardize work to ensure the most efficient outcome possible for an organization and its stakehold-ers.[9] Regulations that guide bureaucratic work, such as development of job descriptions and use of grant funding, are designed to prevent or mitigate the influence of factors like politics, self-interest, mismanage-ment, nepotism, and other issues that might create dysfunction in a civil service system that has the public good as its goal. Public processes, like rule-making, are designed to prevent capricious change, to protect public servants and the public, and to ensure transparency in decision-making. But they take time, require processes, and can get in the way of important, rapid action to address public health.

The sometimes-slow pace of change in government is built into its operating system with the best intentions. But ossification of regulations and their emphasis on control and standardization versus innovation, creativity, and adaptation may stymie agencies and push staff toward management rather than vision-setting and strategy development, which are the core work of leadership. Inflexible work rules, programmatic silos, and categorical funding reinforce the rational, specialized, functional assignment of work and the importance of managing projects versus leading teams and organizations toward a common vision. Management factors often engineer collaboration and alignment out of the system as teams focus on vertical silos and approvals as opposed to horizontal priorities and collective achievement of agency goals. In short, "every system is perfectly designed to get the results it gets."[10] Unfortunately, in some agencies, the system may be delivering less health at greater cost than in other developed nations, sustaining wide disparities and inequities in health and contributing to declining life expectancy.[8]

Public Health 3.0 describes the role of public health leaders as community chief health strategists.[11] Public Health 3.0 calls on governmental public health agencies to engage in "vibrant"[8] cross-sector partnerships; to produce timely, actionable data for health decision-making; and to support blending and braiding of categorical funding to leverage resources and obtain optimal health and well-being. In many governmental public health agencies, the Public Health 3.0 "call to action" clashes with what managers have been told to do for their entire career: to become subject-matter specialists and to advance in the agency as technical leads and experts. The challenges for leaders in a Public Health 3.0 future are: (1) to enable transformation of their agency through evolution and adaptation, (2) to manage the pushback and dissonance that result from change, (3) to propose regulatory and policy changes that support the operational realignments needed, and, ultimately, (4) to more actively, innovatively, and creatively meet the public health needs of their communities. Very few of these challenges rely on technical skills; all rely on strategic skills, especially change management, persuasive communication, policy engagement, and systems thinking.

In a prior commentary on public health leadership and management,[12] it was noted that if practitioners are to realize the promise

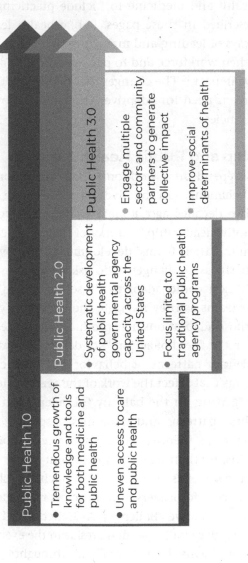

Figure 8.1. The evolution of public health practice. Source: DeSalvo, Karen B. et al. "Public Health 3.0: A Call to Action for Public Health to Meet the Challenges of the 21st Century." *Preventing Chronic Disease* vol. 14 E78. Sep. 7, 2017, doi:10.5888/pcd14.170017. Redrawn with permission.

Public Health 1.0
- Tremendous growth of knowledge and tools for both medicine and public health
- Uneven access to care and public health

Public Health 2.0
- Systematic development of public health governmental agency capacity across the United States
- Focus limited to traditional public health agency programs

Public Health 3.0
- Engage multiple sectors and community partners to generate collective impact
- Improve social determinants of health

Late 1800s

1988 IOM
The Future of Public Health report

Recession

Affordable Care Act

2012 IOM
For the Public's Health reports

of Public Health 3.0, the public health workforce will have to significantly change and adapt. These changes include expanding public health practice beyond the technical and scientific expertise that characterizes public health and medicine to include practicing the nine strategic skills described in these pages. Public health leaders need to develop new ways of leading and managing that better position leaders to engage their workforce and to partner with communities to achieve collective impact.[12] The changes that Public Health 3.0 requires suggest the urgent need for adaptive leadership in governmental public health agencies.

Adaptive Leadership and Public Health 3.0

Public health agencies depend on a workforce that can respond to complex and "vexing"[8] challenges in the diverse and disparate communities they serve. Two decades ago, Ronald Heifetz and Donald Laurie wrote about adaptive leadership,[5,13] a model that casts leaders as individuals who facilitate their teams' development of innovative solutions to complex business challenges, who ask tough questions about how the organization could adapt to those challenges, and who then support their teams as they navigate the uncertainty, distress, and change that those adaptations may produce. The leader role involves looking up from the "field of action,"[5] or day-to-day work of the organization, to identify patterns of behavior and interactions among the various systems that affect the work of the agency. Heifetz and Laurie called this "getting on the balcony."[5] Leaders then help their teams analyze these patterns and dynamics, respond to the adaptive challenges they raise, identify the changes needed for success, and motivate and inspire their teams to implement them.

Rather than defining the leader as technical expert or chief problem-solver, adaptive leadership calls for leaders to work across the organization to identify and resolve adaptive challenges. As Heifetz and Laurie wrote, "the solutions to adaptive challenges don't reside in the executive suite. Solving them requires the involvement of people throughout your organization."[5] Dismissing leadership that emphasizes the leader's role as technical expert or problem-solver as "bankrupt," the authors suggested that leadership requires a move away from leader-as-authority-figure and toward leader-as-provocateur, who helps identify the complicated issues an organization faces and then facilitates collective thinking around adaptations to them.[5]

Public Health 3.0 makes explicit the breadth and complexity of issues that characterize contemporary public health practice. The issues are adaptive challenges and include the decline in U.S. life expectancy and persistent race and ethnic disparities in health outcomes.[8] Adaptive leadership aligns well with the challenges presented by contemporary public health practice and the volatile, uncertain, complex, and ambiguous (VUCA)[14] nature of healthcare policy and public health practice. Even with an increasingly VUCA set of health challenges, such as COVID-19, many public health agencies still emphasize the administrative and operational business of the organization and its programs. This focus on management work is Public Health 2.0 practice that fails to meet the adaptive challenges and to implement the needed changes called for by Public Health 3.0.

Why an Emphasis on Management in Public Health Practice?

In his article "What Leaders Really Do," John Kotter writes, "most U.S. corporations today are overmanaged and underled."[15] This may be true in public-sector agencies as well. Management work, especially financial operations and human resources functions—such as how to hire, how to contract, how to allocate resources— can take up a great deal of a leader's time. Day-to-day operations of an agency are all-consuming: emails need to be read, budgets need to be balanced, staff need to be appraised and directed, information needs to be shared, grants need to be managed, reports need to be filed, data need to be analyzed. Legislative inquiries and compliance and audit functions require careful administrative oversight lest mistakes be made that create negative headlines for an agency that must retain the public's trust.

Management work is essential. In his 2014 commentary on the differences between leadership and management in public health, Dr. Edward L. Baker, former assistant U.S. Surgeon General, noted that "vision without operations and tactics is simply a hallucination."[4]

That is to say, leadership without a solid operation to support it will not succeed. The need for an operational foundation, and the need to minimize risk in a governmental public health department, draw the workforce toward management functions. But a focus on management over leadership makes prioritizing strategic discussions, achieving alignment, and considering organizational positioning extremely difficult. Extending Kotter's insight, it is not surprising that many public health agencies may be overmanaged and underled, because the work of dealing with adaptive challenges is hard, can be uncomfortable, and requires making decisions amid ambiguity and uncertainty. These challenges, however, should not preclude public health practitioners from investing time in both leadership and management.

Responding to, and positioning for, adaptive challenges requires change, and change presents considerable leadership challenges.[16] Adaptive leaders should anticipate questions from their teams like "What grant do we use for that?" "What if my bargaining unit doesn't allow that?" or "What if our intended changes don't work?" The discomfort caused by change can unsettle agency staff and policymakers. Leaders should be able to answer questions, including, "What if my job has to change or my job is not needed?" "What if we have to modernize a statute or write new policy?" or "What if this ends up in a political minefield?" Adaptive leadership requires strategic—not technical—skills, with an eye toward change and transformation. When leading through change, anticipate follower concerns like "I'm not sure I can do that" or "I wasn't trained to do that," or the perennial "That's not my job." Because so much energy is required to push adaptive change forward, to function as community chief health strategist and catalyst, and to mitigate the issues that adapting and transforming may create within teams, public health leadership can be in short supply.

Business writer Alan Deutschman popularized the saying "change or die" with a book of the same title.[17] Too dramatic? Here is an application to public health: change or become irrelevant to the community your agency serves. Indeed, public health competes for relevance in communities where many of the core functions and essential services of public health are now performed by nonprofit organizations, hospitals, and health systems, not governmental public health agencies. Public health managers say they do not have the budgets, the workforce, or the political support to change. Public health leaders see those barriers as challenges to be dealt with, rather than as limiting factors that stifle adaptation, and as factors that can be overcome.

Balancing Leadership and Management

Adaptive leadership is a model for advancing the public health leader's role as strategist and catalyst. Public health practice requires integrating leadership and management and consciously reflecting on time spent in both areas. The duality of leading and managing in public health is shown in figure 8.2, which is based on the Chinese principle of yin and yang. The principle describes how two opposing forces, often working at contrary purposes, are interrelated and interdependent. Management and leadership are complementary functions, necessary parts of public health practice. The focus to date of governmental public health practice has been on management; Public Health 3.0 suggests that the future of public health requires greater emphasis on strategy and leadership.

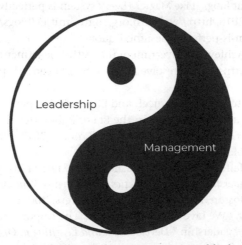

Figure 8.2. Balancing leadership and management in public health practice.

References

1. Paul J. H. Schoemaker, Steve Krupp, and Samantha Howland, "Strategic Leadership: The Essential Skills," *Harvard Business Review* January/February (2013): 1–5.
2. John W. Gardner, *On Leadership* (New York: The Free Press, 1990), 3.
3. Peter M. Senge, *The Fifth Discipline: The Art & Practice of the Learning Organization* (London: Doubleday, 2006).
4. Edward L. Baker, "Leadership and Management—Guiding Principles, Best Practices, and Core Attributes," *Journal of Public Health Management and Practice* 20, no. 3 (2014): 356–357, https://journals.lww.com/jphmp/fulltext/2014/05000/leadership_and_management_guiding_princip les,_best.15.aspx.
5. Ronald A. Heifetz and Donald L. Laurie, "The Work of Leadership," *Harvard Business Review* December (2001): 1–13. Reprint #R0111K.
6. Richard L. Hughes, Katherine C. Beatty, and D. L. Dinwoodie, *Becoming a Strategic Leader: Your Role in Your Organization's Enduring Success*, (San Francisco, CA: Jossey-Bass, 2014).
7. Vineet Nayar, "Three Differences Between Managers and Leaders," *Harvard Business Review* August (2013), https://hbr.org/2013/08/tests-of-a-leadership-transiti.
8. Office of the Assistant Secretary for Health, U.S. Department of Health and Human Services, *Public Health 3.0: A Call to Action to Create a 21st Century Public Health Infrastructure* (Washington, DC: US DHHS, 2016).
9. Tony Waters and Dagmar Waters, *Weber's Rationalism and Modern Society: New Translations on Politics, Bureaucracy, and Social Stratification* (New York: Palgrave Macmillan, 2016).
10. Improvement Blog, "Like Magic? (Every system is perfectly designed . . .)," August 15, 2015, http://www.ihi.org/communities/blogs/origin-of-every-system-is-perfectly-designed-quote.
11. "The High Achieving Governmental Health Department in 2020," RESOLVE, https://www.resolve.ngo/site-healthleadershipforum/hd2020.htm.
12. Michael Fraser, Brian Castrucci, and Elizabeth Harper, "Public Health Leadership and Management in the Era of Public Health 3.0," *Journal of Public Health Management and Practice* 23, no. 1 (2017): 90–92, https://pubmed.ncbi.nlm.nih.gov/27870719/.
13. Ronald A. Heifetz, Alexander Grashow, and Marty Linsky, *The Practice of Adaptive Leadership: Tools and Tactics for Changing Your Organization and the World* (Boston, MA: Harvard Business Press, 2009).
14. Anita Sarkar, "We Live in a VUCA World: The Importance of Responsible Leadership," *Development and Learning in Organizations* 30, no. 3 (2016): 9–12, https://www.researchgate.net/publicat

ion/303317070_We_live_in_a_VUCA_World_the_importance_of_res ponsible_leadership.

15. John P. Kotter, "What Leaders Really Do," *Harvard Business Review* December (2001): 1–12. Reprint #R0111F, p. 3.

16. John P. Kotter, *Leading Change* (Boston, MA: Harvard Business Review Press, 2012).

17. Alan Deutschman, *Change or Die: The Three Keys to Change at Work and in Life* (New York: Harper, 2008).

9

STRATEGIC SKILLS IN FOCUS:
- ▶ *Systems and Strategic Thinking*
- ▶ *Resource Management*
- ▶ *Data-Driven Decision-Making*

Problem-Solving and Decision-Making Skills for Public Health Practice

MICHAEL R. FRASER

PEOPLE FACE MYRIAD PROBLEMS AND make countless decisions every day. In the first hours of the day, individuals problem-solve and make decisions they may not even be conscious of, such as when to get up, what to wear, what to eat for breakfast, or whether to have a second cup of coffee. Most everyday decisions are relatively inconsequential and straightforward, requiring minor effort and little collaboration. Larger problems and more important decisions, on the other hand, require prolonged attention, greater deliberation, and the input and expertise of others. These may include problems and decisions like how to balance a program's budget, how to evaluate a prevention campaign, how to increase community engagement around contact tracing and testing for COVID-19, or finding the best use of new technology to improve laboratory reporting. Effectively solving problems like these and reaching the best decisions when the outcomes are consequential are the focus of this chapter.

Michael R. Fraser, *Problem-Solving and Decision-Making Skills for Public Health Practice* In: *Building Strategic Skills for Better Health: A Primer for Public Health Professionals*. Edited by: Michael R. Fraser and Brian C. Castrucci, Oxford University Press. © de Beaumont Foundation 2024. DOI: 10.1093/oso/9780197744604.003.0010

What Is the Problem with Problem-Solving?

Why is problem-solving a skill desired by so many managers and supervisors and significant enough to be one of just nine strategic skills for public health practice? In short, employees who can effectively solve complex problems generate exceptional value for an organization by bringing innovative and creative solutions to organizational challenges. Such employees are often easier to manage because their ability to problem-solve may mean they require less hands-on supervision. Effective problem-solvers are often more engaged in their work because they can brainstorm and work collaboratively to develop solutions. They may be more likely to succeed at work in an era that requires adaptability and strategic thinking. A study of U.S. educators and policymakers found that 85% of those surveyed considered creative problem-solving a critical skill for students to learn; 84% of educators and 68% of policymakers, however, said there was not enough emphasis on creative problem-solving in American education.[1] Lack of formal training in problem-solving means that while some public health practitioners may be fluent in these approaches, many have never spent much time thinking about what problem-solving means or how to go about solving the problems we face, especially the complex and seemingly intractable ones that confront public health. One of the more comprehensive definitions of problem-solving describes it as "the act of defining a problem; determining the cause of the problem; identifying, prioritizing, and selecting alternatives for a solution; and implementing a solution."[2] The parts of this definition, and the definition in Table 9.1, are significant: problem-solving is a process, not a single act; there are multiple solutions to be identified and considered; and the preferred solution has to be selected, effectively implemented, and then monitored and evaluated.

Effective problem-solving can take lots of work, especially for complex problems with no right answer. However, the costs of not solving a problem are high, due to potentially having to solve the problem later and invest additional time and team resources. As such, skilled problem-solvers are important assets in any organization. Unskilled or over-skilled use of problem-solving competencies by an employee,

Table 9.1. Seven Decision-Making Styles, Vroom-Yetten Decision Tree Model

---

Autocratic 1 (A1): You solve the problem or make the decision yourself, using information available at the time.

Autocratic 2 (A2): You obtain information from others and then yourself decide on the solution. You may or may not share what problem you are trying to solve—the role for others is to get you information, not to provide solutions or to help make the decision. (Individual or group problem)

Consultative 1 (C1): You share the problem with others, asking individuals for their ideas and suggestions but not bringing them together as a group. Then you make the decision, which may or may not reflect their input. (Individual or group problem)

For individual problems—problems that involve you as a leader or an individual on your team	*For group problems—problems that involve a group of people, a team, or an organization*
Group 1 (G1): You explain the problem to one of your subordinates and exchange information and ideas about it. You both contribute to resolving the problem.	Delegative 1 (D1): You delegate the problem to someone else, providing information that you possess but giving him or her responsibility for solving the problem independently. The decision has your full support.
Consultative 2 (C2): You share the problem with others in a group meeting and ask for input on solutions. During this meeting, you reach the decision, which may or may not include the contributions of others.	Group 2 (G2): You share the problem with others as a group. Together you generate and evaluate alternatives and attempt to reach consensus about a solution. Your role is to facilitate the meeting, not to influence the group to adopt your solution. The decision of the group has your full support.

Sources: Adapted from "The Vroom-Yetten Decision Model: Deciding How to Decide," MindTools,[10] and John A. Wagner and John R. Hollenbeck, *Organizational Behavior: Securing Competitive Advantage*,[11] pp. 253–254.

however, can slow down organizational momentum, waste resources, or keep staff from meeting agency goals.[3]

Approaches to Problem-Solving

Faced with complex problems in uncertain environments, many professionals, especially those with extensive experience in their fields, rely almost solely on instinct and prior observations. This can be a successful approach to problem-solving. However, overreliance on experience and expertise has disadvantages: Prior observations can blind problem-solvers to new and different solutions to problems. Another disadvantage of relying on one's "gut" or hunch may be the sacrifice of trusting one's "head" or using more analytical methods, data, or evidence to solve a problem. Using a combination of head and gut can lead to more effective problem-solving (especially when combined with the right decision-making process, described below). This is not to discount the importance of familiarity, experience, instinct, and intuition in solving problems. Rather, it is important to realize those same positive traits can limit creativity or innovation when a problem is not what it first seems to be, or the environment has changed since earlier solutions were developed. In "A Brief History of Decision Making," Buchanan and O'Connell write:

> Of course the gut/brain dichotomy is largely false. Few decision makers ignore good information when they can get it. And most accept that there will be times they can't get it and so will have to rely on instinct. Fortunately, the intellect informs both intuition and analysis, and research shows that people's instincts are often quite good.[4]

Perhaps the biggest problem with problem-solving is that many people are charged with a rush to get started and then solve the wrong problem. Here are two examples from public health practice:

- Volume at a public health agency's immunization clinic was down and the school year was about to begin. The program administrator believed the problem was a lack of community knowledge about the clinic and paid for radio, online, and print advertising to inform the public about the clinic's availability. The program administrator's conclusion was not based in evidence or information, however. The administrator did not consider that clinic hours were from 9 a.m. to noon, when most parents are working, and may have wasted valuable resources deploying a solution for the wrong problem. Focus groups of parents conducted in partnership with the local school system found that it was clinic hours, not community knowledge, at issue. Vaccination rates went up after clinic hours changed so that parents could stop by before work.

- A disease investigator noticed that while the number of cases was small, congenital syphilis cases in her community were increasing, especially among women seen at a particular hospital. She decided to work with her agency's STD team to present a "grand rounds" session about congenital syphilis to educate the hospital's medical staff about the state requirement that pregnant women be tested at a prenatal visit during each trimester. After the training, rates continued to increase—the grand rounds solution solved the wrong problem. The correct problem to address was provider stigmatization of STDs. Some hospital clinicians assumed that many of their patients were not at risk or the clinicians did not want to discuss STDs with patients and thought that patients with an STD should be seen elsewhere. When staff addressed the problem of stigma, shared data on risk in the population served by the clinic, and addressed perceptions of STDs among providers and staff, cases of congenital syphilis declined.

These examples demonstrate the value of asking "Are we solving the right problem?" early in the process, especially when responding to a new problem or when there is great uncertainty. Spending time to accurately define a problem is a critical first step. As Wedell-Wedellsborg suggests, most companies may think they are good at problem-solving, but they are not so great at defining the true problem to be solved.[5]

Rational, data-driven, and evidence-informed approaches to identifying and solving problems are common in public health practice. Public health professionals use volumes of assessment results, surveillance data, and community input to help determine and solve public health problems. The data instruct future action, ascertain potential needs, and help clarify the issues to be solved. Rational problem-solving approaches like these are common in quality improvement, especially when incremental or iterative changes are needed and can easily be evaluated before and after solution implementation. The rational approach is also helpful when the solution set to a problem is relatively well understood and can be translated into recommendations for evidence-based public health action. Figure 9.1 summarizes a general process for rational problem-solving developed by the American Society for Quality.

Organic approaches to problem-solving examine adaptive or strategic solutions rather than linear or technical ones. Organic approaches are shaped by inquiry and discussions of possibilities and opportunities, not deficits. The adaptive approach seeks solutions that might not be easily analyzed with data or may not have potential solutions that can easily be weighted, rated, or even be considered optimal because of a problem's complexity. In an organic approach, solutions may not be identified until conversation and discovery of various perspectives are raised, considered, and shared. Solutions using an organic approach are the result of dialogue and imagination, not re-engineering or repair.

Appreciative inquiry (AI) is one example of an organic approach.[6] AI asserts that problems may be the result of individual perspectives and perceptions or the way we look at something we take as a given. Therefore, deep inquiry is needed to understand an issue before developing a solution or recommendations for change. [7,8] The 4-D

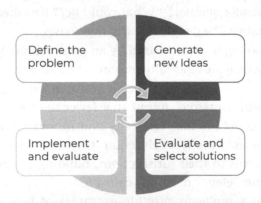

Define the problem

Generate new Ideas

Implement and evaluate

Evaluate and select solutions

Figure 9.1. Example of a general problem-solving process. ASQ, the American Society for Quality, describes four steps in their problem-solving approach:[2] (1) Define the problem. (2) Generate new ideas. (3) Evaluate and select solutions. (4) Implement and evaluate. Source: *What Is Problem Solving?* ASQ, https://asq.org/quality-resources/problem-solving. Redrawn with permission.

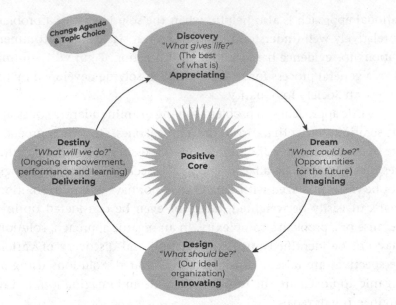

Figure 9.2. 4-D cycle of appreciative inquiry. Source: Whitney, Diana, and Amanda Trosten-Bloom. *The Power of Appreciative Inquiry: A Practical Guide to Positive Change.* Berret-Koehler, 2010.[6] Redrawn with permission.

cycle (figure 9.2) used in the AI approach seeks to question those perceptions and givens (the discovery and appreciation phase), "appreciating" or acknowledging the perspectives we bring to our work and asking the broader question, "What could be?" (the dream phase) to adapt and change (the design and destiny phases).

Problem-solving is characterized by an emphasis on creativity and innovation, which are especially important when working with complex problems. Unfortunately, recent research on the governmental public health workforce found that fewer than half of all public health workers believe that creativity and innovation are rewarded in their agencies.[9] To effectively equip the public health workforce to solve problems in their jurisdictions, building the creativity and innovation competency of staff is called for.

Two complex problems provide examples of how rational and organic approaches could be applied in practice. First, how should public health agencies adapt and even compete with hospital and health-system initiatives that focus on population health improvement and related programs to address the social determinants of health as part of federal incentives to implement value-based healthcare? One technical (or rational) solution is to continue to support public health programs that focus on prevention and community health but to solve the need to adapt by iterating or building on existing programs and collaborating with healthcare organizations to move "upstream" toward addressing a community's social needs. An adaptive (or organic) solution is to design completely new and different programs and services that play to the strengths of various institutions or stakeholders, working first to imagine necessary systems to produce health at the community level rather than trying to iterate on existing work. This would require eliminating formerly critical services that are no longer relevant or engaging the populations served by the healthcare and public health systems in different ways to co-create opportunities for promoting wellness. An adaptive solution may dramatically reshape what the health department does with hospital partners. Here, rational and organic problem-solving are quite different approaches to the same problem.

The second example looks at efforts by federal, state, and local agencies to improve the speed and accuracy of communicable disease surveillance by modernizing the information technology systems used by governmental public health agencies. These agencies seek to improve how healthcare and public health data are shared within and between states, and between states and the federal government. Existing fragmented, legacy disease-reporting systems, outdated IT infrastructure, and restrictive data-use policies governing patient privacy and data-sharing are important issues to address, as is the need for investments in technology infrastructure at all levels of government. One technical solution is to use existing state data systems and to create new interstate "gateways" to share data between states, and to revise or approve new policies for sharing data that build on existing systems and streamline reporting. Indeed, this is what state and national partners have done to share Prescription Drug Monitoring Program (PDMP) data more efficiently using federal dollars appropriated by the U.S. Congress.

An adaptive solution is to examine and appreciate how various sectors have approached similar challenges, engaging new stakeholders in conversations about the problem, and then evolving a solution with new information and different partners that creates new ways for data to be reported, aggregated, and shared. The rational approach focuses on re-engineering and iteration; the organic method focuses on adaptive challenges that incorporate both new thinkers and new thinking to solve the problem. Each will lead to a solution, but in this example the adaptive approach may be the more lasting one, although it could require more time and resources for visioning, stakeholder engagement, and the research and inquiry processes.

Effective Decision-making Processes: Make Decision Maker Bias Explicit

Decision-making refers to the process by which someone assesses options and selects a course of action. Imagine you are a supervisor faced with a fairly straightforward decision: how to rate an employee on her annual evaluation. You might consider factors like the quality of her work, her achievement of goals against agency benchmarks, and perhaps a measure of teamwork or collaboration with others in the department. You follow your agency's standard process, complete the forms, and meet with the employee to share feedback, ultimately deciding to rate her "excellent," which results in a 3% salary increase for outstanding performance.

What may be hard to see in the process described above are the cognitive biases and perceptions that went into your decision. Perhaps you socialize with this employee, have established a friendship, and want to rank her highly to avoid an awkward discussion away from work. Perhaps you know she works just as hard as the other employees your peers rate as "excellent" and want to establish this employee's equal standing with others in the same category, even if she fell short on a few of the tasks you assigned her. Perhaps you have supervised this employee for many years, have given her the top rating every year, and know she would be let down not to be rated as highly as last year despite a few stumbles in performance.

This scenario touches on a few cognitive biases, which are part of nearly all human decision-making. Cognitive biases can be helpful, especially when we need to make quick or multiple decisions in a short period of time. For example, are you inside a burning house? Run outside and dial 911. There is no need to remain inside and determine all possible options. Assessing every factor involved in a decision every time we make one could become paralyzing. So that we do not have to think consciously and explicitly about every decision, our minds create heuristics, or mental shortcuts, that help us select an action more quickly and easily. Heuristics, however, may keep us from considering better options precisely because they are shortcuts and, because of the way our minds work, may limit the range of actions we recognize based on prior experience.

Some common heuristics that get in the way of effective decision-making are:

- *Action bias*: the tendency to favor action over inaction. Making any decision is considered better than making no decision at all, even if more analysis is needed or taking no action is the best course of action.
- *Anchoring bias*: paying greatest attention to the first sources of information ("anchors") you gather in your decision-making process. Anchor information is given more weight than information gathered subsequently.
- *Authority bias*: attributing greater weight to the opinion or point of view of an authority figure or someone with influence in evaluating or selecting a course of action, although it may not be the best option.
- *Confirmation bias*: selectively using evidence that supports your position or point of view as confirmation of your beliefs. We are more likely to look for and find evidence that supports our beliefs than to identify alternatives and to select a course of action that requires different beliefs.
- *Conformity bias*: the tendency to think like the people around you when reaching a decision rather than stating or developing a different or unique position. We may select a course of action to obtain consensus or avoid conflict.

- *Halo bias* or *"halo effect"*: making positive judgments about people based on an initial impression of one characteristic and extending those positive judgments to everything about them.
- *Status quo bias*: reaching a decision that supports the current state versus an ideal or different state. Actions remain consistent with how things have always been.
- *Sunk-cost bias*: remaining with a course of action because you are invested in it, although it might not be the best choice.

Given all the information we must process to make a decision, we use shortcuts to efficiently move forward. It is next to impossible to eliminate cognitive bias—if we could, we would be overwhelmed by considering all the factors that influence a decision and would perhaps fail to act. Eliminating bias, however, is not the goal; instead, bias should be made explicit. Acknowledge and discuss it, then work to address it along with the other factors under consideration.

In the employee evaluation example, the supervisor could have discussed his ratings with another supervisor, ensuring that he was being objective in giving the employee her 3% increase and "outstanding" rating for the year. The organization could address some biases by convening supervisors before finalizing reviews, by calibrating ratings together, by discussing work outcomes, by confirming that supervisors would rate their employees similarly given specific situations, and by making biases known (confronting the halo effect). A good decision-making process recognizes biases and addresses them as part of deliberations.

Deciding How to Decide

Beyond considering the heuristics that are part of decision-making, organizations need to examine how they reach decisions, particularly those made by leadership. Many people use dominance as a decision-making style in every case, no matter how consequential the issue. An agency head may always use her authority to make decisions, even those that would best be delegated to senior leaders. Staff may desire to be part of decision-making, especially if it pertains to work culture or employee benefits, but autocratic decision makers may fail to consult with others because they believe they have all the information needed, no matter the topic.

Victor Vroom and Philip Yetton designed an eight-question decision tree to help leaders arrive at the right style for making a decision.[10] The model describes seven styles that characterize decision-making (see table 9.1) and points to when leaders should reach a decision on their own (autocratic or authoritarian decision-making), when to consult with others (consultative decision-making), when to give decision-making authority to a subordinate (delegative decision-making), and when to step aside and give decision-making authority to a group (group-based or collaborative decision-making). The eight questions move decision makers along a path toward the style appropriate for a given circumstance. The questions are:

1. If the decision were accepted, would it make a difference which course of action was adopted?
2. Do I have sufficient information to reach a high-quality decision?
3. Do subordinates have sufficient additional information to result in a high-quality decision?
4. Do I know exactly what information is needed, who possesses it, and how to collect it?
5. Is acceptance of the decision by my subordinates critical to effective implementation?
6. If I were to make the decision myself, is it certain that it would be accepted by subordinates?
7. Can subordinates be trusted to base solutions on organizational considerations?
8. Is conflict among subordinates likely in preferred solutions?

Answering Yes or No to each of the above guides the decision maker toward one of the seven decision styles.

The Vroom-Yetten model will be of interest to agency staff who want to learn about how leadership engages others in making decisions, when leadership makes decisions on its own, and when leadership will delegate or allow employee groups to make decisions. The transparency that arises from a discussion of decision-making styles and how they are used can help build buy-in for agency decisions of all kinds, even those that do not include staff input.

Avoiding Groupthink

A significant problem in decision-making is groupthink.[12] Broadly defined, groupthink occurs when a group comes to a premature consensus on a course of action before all options are considered. Groupthink prevents effective decision-making by failing to allow ample discussion, shutting down creative conflict or disagreement on issues, and limiting consideration of various factors that should be examined.[4] If constructive disagreement is not raised for fear of creating conflict or upsetting the owner of a chosen decision, or because the leader is not invested in learning from the perspectives of others, the goal of agreement overrides the goal of reaching the best decision. Groupthink is a problem in organizations where teams are homogeneous in thought or perspective and in conflict-averse organizations where disagreement is considered insubordinate and unproductive.

One way to counter groupthink is to diversify the group making the decision. A diverse group, managed and facilitated well, may raise more varied perspectives and opinions than a homogeneous group and is likely to avoid premature consensus so long as the process encourages eliciting those options. Another tactic is to purposefully push for dissent and disagreement in any group that seems to be reaching agreement too quickly.[12] Consider designating a "strategic dissenter"[13] to raise tough questions and offer alternatives as a devil's advocate in the decision-making process. Constructive conflict around decision-making leads to better decisions, while premature consensus or collective adoption of an idea leads to poorer ones. Generally, this is because important alternatives and points of view are not given thought in a process that emphasizes agreement over divergence. Premature agreement can undermine a decision, erode engagement and motivation, and hinder buy-in by agency staff.

Summary

Problems are solved and decisions are made daily by every employee in every organization. While the scope and impact of decisions vary, it is important to intentionally consider how decisions are made, especially by organizational leaders, what biases are at play, and how to make those biases explicit and avoid the pitfalls of leaving them unchecked. Steering clear of groupthink—a pattern that may leave certain perspectives or ideas unrecognized—is also important when a team makes decisions. Identifying a strategic dissenter and discussing what kinds of decision-making approaches to use for various types of decisions are evidence-based ways to address biases in your organization.

Identifying the right problem to solve and considering the best approach to solving it enhances problem-solving. Rushing to a solution or taking too long to analyze options can stymie a team. Creativity and innovation are important for solving complex problems, but research on the public health workforce finds these skills underutilized in governmental public health agencies nationwide. Effective problem-solving involves both intuition and experience, as well as consideration of data and evidence. Skilled problem-solvers develop multiple solutions to a problem and then discern the best option using data and experience—this saves valuable management time and efficiently utilizes the resources of an organization.

Problem-solving and decision-making are two things we do all day, every day, yet consideration of how to reach good decisions receives little attention in most organizations. Public health practitioners who understand how to raise issues and options before taking action, make biases explicit, and prize creativity and innovation in solving complex problems or making difficult decisions create value for their organizations and ultimately generate better health for the communities they serve.

References

1. "Creative Problem Solving," Adobe Systems Incorporated, January 2018, http://cps.adobeeducate.com/.
2. "What Is Problem Solving?" American Society for Quality, https://asq.org/quality-resources/problem-solving.

3. Michael M. Lombardo and Robert W. Eichinger, *FYI For Your Improvement*, 4th ed. (Minneapolis, MN: Lominger International, 2006).
4. Leigh Buchanan and Andrew O'Connell, "A Brief History of Decision Making," *Harvard Business Review* January (2006), https://hbr.org/2006/01/a-brief-history-of-decision-making.
5. Thomas Wedell-Wedellsborg, "Are You Solving the Right Problems?" *Harvard Business Review* January (2017), https://hbr.org/2017/01/are-you-solving-the-right-problems.
6. Diana Whitney and Amanda Trosten-Bloom, *The Power of Appreciative Inquiry: A Practical Guide to Positive Change* (San Francisco, CA: Berrett-Koehler Publishers, 2010).
7. Francesca Gino, "When Solving Problems, Think About What You Could Do, Not What You Should Do," *Harvard Business Review* April (2018), https://hbr.org/2018/04/when-solving-problems-think-about-what-you-could-do-not-what-you-should-do.
8. Carter McNamara, "Appreciative Inquiry," https://managementhelp.org/businessresearch/appreciative-inquiry.htm.
9. Rachel Locke et al., "Unleashing the Creativity and Innovation of Our Greatest Resource—The Governmental Public Health Workforce," *Journal of Public Health Management and Practice* 25, suppl. 2 (2019): S96–S102, https://pubmed.ncbi.nlm.nih.gov/30720622/.
10. "The Vroom-Yetton Decision Model: Deciding How to Decide," MindTools, https://www.mindtools.com/pages/article/newTED_91.htm.
11. John A. Wagner and John R. Hollenbeck, *Organizational Behavior: Securing Competitive Advantage*, 2nd ed. (New York: Routledge, 2015).
12. Art Markham, "The Problem-Solving Process That Prevents Groupthink," *Harvard Business Review* November (2015), https://hbr.org/2015/11/the-problem-solving-process-that-prevents-groupthink.
13. Torben Emmerling and Duncan Rooders, "7 Strategies for Better Group Decision-Making," *Harvard Business Review* September (2020), https://hbr.org/2020/09/7-strategies-for-better-group-decision-making.

10

Purpose, Passion, and the Public's Health

A Brief Guide to Employee Motivation and Engagement for Public Health Leaders and Managers

AMBER NORRIS WILLIAMS, MICHAEL R. FRASER, AND ROBIN MATTHIES

GOVERNMENTAL PUBLIC HEALTH AGENCIES RELY on a well-trained, motivated, and engaged workforce to protect and promote the health of people and communities. When employees are motivated and engaged at work, they feel enthusiastic about their work, contribute at higher levels, and seek more work to advance their organization's mission. Engaged employees—who are both involved in their work and committed to their organization's goals—have multiple benefits for employers. Employee engagement is linked to lower absenteeism, higher employee retention, higher productivity, higher-quality work, and better customer service. Sadly, many workers are not fully engaged at work, including those working in governmental public health agencies.

Amber Norris Williams, Michael R. Fraser, and Robin Matthies, *Purpose, Passion, and the Public's Health* In: *Building Strategic Skills for Better Health: A Primer for Public Health Professionals.* Edited by: Michael R. Fraser and Brian C. Castrucci, Oxford University Press. © de Beaumont Foundation 2024. DOI: 10.1093/oso/9780197744604.003.0011

Public health agencies are facing two critical moments: the COVID-19 pandemic and the national reckoning on racial inequity. COVID-19 highlights the vital services provided by the public health workforce to the communities they serve. In the decade leading up to the pandemic, the governmental public health workforce saw significant job losses despite national warnings and calls for greater investments.[1] These cuts have both hampered the ability of public health agencies to quickly respond to the pandemic and have negatively impacted employee morale and engagement as staff work longer hours, face increased public scrutiny and criticism for public health mitigation efforts, and worry for their own health and well-being. The Center for State and Local Government Excellence (SLGE) notes a significant increase in employee burnout and fatigue among state and local employees, including public health agency staff.[2]

In addition, the national reckoning on racism and racial injustice has had a significant impact on governmental public health agencies. Beyond the work public health agencies do to address the long-term health impacts of racism, there is a need for public health agencies to make systemic changes internally in addressing discrimination, inequity, and exclusion. A significant effort to rebuild the public health workforce is on the agenda of national decision makers; a companion effort to address workforce resilience, including employee motivation and engagement in public health agencies, should also be undertaken. While employee engagement and motivation are important during typical operations, the COVID-19 epidemic illustrates the specific challenge and need to address these factors while also responding to an extended worldwide crisis.

Though governmental agencies face unique and difficult challenges, increasing employee engagement and motivation is within the control and budget of every governmental public health manager and leader. Further, it is imperative in the context of the COVID-19 response. This chapter addresses some of the ways that governmental public health leaders can increase employee engagement and unlock employee motivation by leveraging the important purpose and meaningful work of governmental public health. The chapter also highlights one state's approach to finding "joy in work" in the effort to address burnout and resulting disengagement. The importance of building joy, even during a national emergency like a pandemic, cannot be overstated. Such efforts will yield much higher employee satisfaction, engagement, and commitment to work by promoting resilience, reducing burnout, and demonstrating that agency leadership cares about the health and well-being of its personnel.

Challenges to Workforce Motivation and Engagement

Surveys of the public health workforce and the authors' own observations from working nationally with public health leaders suggest that many governmental public health agencies find it hard to recruit and retain to meet staffing needs. The agencies often face fiscal and statutory barriers to adding positions, changing job titles and employee classifications, increasing salaries, providing bonuses or other financial incentives, and offering benefits like telework or flexible scheduling. Governmental public health leaders report difficulty in recruiting and retaining a highly qualified workforce for a variety of reasons.

Government agencies especially compete for talent with the private sector and nonprofit organizations and find it difficult to compete with those groups on salary. Government agencies regularly face hiring freezes because of budget or political challenges, which can create barriers to recruitment. Other roadblocks reported by health agency leaders include: elimination of, or rollbacks to, some of the traditionally generous healthcare and retirement benefits offered in government; civil service regulations and collective bargaining agreements that can create a lengthy process for selecting and hiring candidates; limited agency resources for professional development and training; prevalent and increasing antigovernment sentiment; and negative perceptions of the public sector.

As described in chapter 1, the 2021 Public Health Workforce Interests and Needs Survey (PH WINS), a national survey of the state and local governmental public health workforce, recently estimated that nearly half of the workforce plans to retire or leave their jobs within the next five years.[3] Agencies pay a high price for turnover. The cost of losing an employee can be as much as twice the employee's salary, considering lost productivity, costs of hiring and onboarding a new employee, and the potential spillover effect to employees who witness high turnover and then disengage.[4] Therefore, public health agencies must address the factors that make their organizations desirable places to work as they recruit new employees and seek to retain current ones.

What Is Employee Engagement? Why Does It Matter?

Underlying most definitions of employee engagement is the importance of employee commitment to an organization's goals and an employee's positive relationships with others. High employee engagement is associated with many positive workplace factors, including lower turnover, greater customer satisfaction, and stronger overall organizational performance.[5] Engagement is not just about individual employees; it also occurs in work teams and across all levels of an organization. Engaged individuals and teams can better obtain, mobilize, and leverage their resources, and engaged employees learn more, are more creative, and have higher levels of enthusiasm and energy than disengaged teams.[6] Engaged employees also invest greater discretionary effort into their work and their organization's mission.

Despite these benefits, national trends show that most of the U.S. workforce is not engaged at work, with only 35% of employees reporting that they are engaged.[7] The cost of low employee engagement in the private sector is striking: Gallup (2013) found that disengaged employees have 37% higher absenteeism, 18% lower productivity, and cost $3,400 for every $10,000 in annual salary; the analysis estimates that the entire cost of disengaged employees to the American economy is $450 billion to $550 billion each year. While there are no estimates of the cost of disengagement in public health agencies, it can be surmised that disengaged employees in government similarly experience high rates of absenteeism and lower productivity. Low "profitability" may result, for example, in fewer improvements in health and well-being in the community an agency serves, or a less coordinated and less effective approach to preventing or mitigating the consequences of a deadly new virus.

However, PH WINS data also suggest that individuals working in governmental public health at the state and local levels are more engaged than the average American worker. Measures from the survey illustrate that the governmental public health workforce is highly dedicated to its work (94% of respondents reported that they are "determined to give their best effort at work each day" and 82% reported feeling "completely involved in their work"). These findings suggest high employee commitment and engagement in public health agencies. Considering the benefits of high employee engagement, public health managers can leverage this strength to sustain and advance their organization's mission.

There are many strategies for sustaining and increasing employee engagement. Because engagement is highly correlated with employees' relationships with their supervisors,[8] agencies should look at how they select, train, and develop supervisors to ensure that they have positive relationships with their teams. Agencies can consider training for new and seasoned managers to build skills and to emphasize the importance of their role in sustaining and increasing engagement. In addition, because commitment is linked to an employee's identification with the mission of an organization, agencies can spotlight "mission moments" for their teams through public acknowledgment, kudos, and staff appreciation. These moments can include recognition of how an employee or team lived their organization's core values and examples of how the agency made a positive difference in the community. Creating shared identity through team development opportunities, volunteer work, and other "give back" initiatives also can promote engagement, by showing that an agency cares about employees and the community it serves. Box 10.1 summarizes some activities managers can undertake to increase employee engagement.

Motivate Employees by Leveraging Passion and Purpose, Not Just Pay

Closely tied to employee engagement is employee motivation, or what drives an individual to perform at work. Traditionally, organizations have focused on the extrinsic factors that influence individual motivation, such as salary, benefits, recognition, and praise. These

---

BOX 10.1. EXAMPLES OF ENGAGEMENT ACTIVITIES

- Be accessible.
- Share authentic feedback, focused on employee growth and development.
- Coach and teach, rather than chastise and correct.
- Become aware of your own unintentional biases.
- Provide flexibility in work hours or locations (flextime, telework).
- Sponsor team development retreats that emphasize commitment and impact.
- Address stress in the workplace, and work to mitigate unhealthy stress organization-wide.
- Recognize and reward achievement and commitment to the organization.
- Make core values explicit; make the organization's mission "real" to employees with stories of impact.
- Offer professional development and training experiences that help employees learn and grow.
- Engage employees in the work of the organization from the start of their tenure through onboarding, mentoring, and coaching.
- Promote wellness and resilience.
- Encourage experimentation and innovation and allow room for mistakes.
- Strengthen communication between leadership and all employees.
- Promote sharing of successes and acknowledge results.
- Ask what would increase employee and team engagement and personalize your efforts to individual staff members.
- Model inclusive behaviors by asking for, encouraging, and listening to feedback from staff at all levels.

---

are external rewards that influence an individual's performance at work. Pay, promotions, and other material benefits do not necessarily increase employee motivation, particularly for any significant length of time. Leaders and managers must focus on addressing the role of intrinsic motivation for organizational success and creation of a high-performing organization.

Intrinsic motivators are the factors internal to individuals that drive their performance and commitment. These include an employee's desire to learn at work, to grow and develop as an individual, to do meaningful work, and to find purpose at work. Motivated employees are more efficient, are more likely to focus on their own development and growth, and have lower absenteeism. While organizational cultures are changing, many legacy human resource systems are based on addressing employees' extrinsic motivation (pay, promotion, praise) with less attention to intrinsic motivation (purpose, passion, progress/growth). A focus of contemporary organizational development approaches is how to make work a place where employees find purpose and meaning and not just a paycheck. Very few individuals go into public health seeking high pay or praise, suggesting that most practitioners value their work and the difference public health makes in their communities.

Effective managers understand that while they cannot force motivation, their most critical role is to create the conditions in which employees can motivate themselves to do their best work. While there is no one right away to motivate and engage employees, and there are distinct constraints related to administrative policies and rules within governmental agencies, it is critical that public health managers and agencies continuously focus on increasing employee enthusiasm and commitment and helping employees find and activate their own intrinsic motivation and drive. Managers have discretion, even within governmental agencies, to address both extrinsic and intrinsic motivation. Successful leaders think about rewards as well as crafting opportunities for employees to grow at work by prioritizing staff development and providing recognition, coaching, and mentorship to employees.

Intrinsically motivated employees desire challenging work, control, or autonomy in the development of work products; recognition of accomplishments; and connections with their supervisor and coworkers. Many jobs in governmental public health allow for intrinsic motivation because much of public health work is complex, challenging, and requires collaboration. Tactics for making jobs even more intrinsically motivating include creating opportunities to expand jobs with new or shared duties to encompass a larger scope of functions or tasks; promoting job rotation, where employees expand their knowledge by working in several positions in the same organization; and enriching jobs by increasing autonomy and direct control of work products.[9] Managers looking to enhance the impact of their teams can leverage intrinsic motivation to strengthen engagement and improve staff resiliency.

Finding Joy in Work at the Wisconsin Department of Health Services

In 2016, the Wisconsin Department of Health Services responded to a call from Wisconsin's first lady to make Wisconsin a trauma-informed state. This effort included key state agencies' learning more about the impact of adverse childhood experiences (ACEs) and adopting practices to build a more trauma-informed workforce. After learning that many staff had experienced significant stressors/traumas professionally and/or personally, a statewide steering committee, led by the public health director, decided to make wellness and resilience efforts a 2018 priority. The state identified project goals that included improving employee engagement and satisfaction, leadership development, and improving staff resiliency. To emphasize the importance of this effort, the public health agency also added trauma-informed workplace efforts to their strategic plan.

Wisconsin's team used two main resources to drive their efforts: The Institute for Healthcare Improvement's (IHI) Framework for Improving Joy in Work[10] and change strategies from Achor's *The Happiness Advantage*.[11] The Joy in Work toolkit was developed to address clinical burnout in healthcare settings, and it details factors that can improve morale and satisfaction at work; Achor's book shares findings from positive psychology and focuses on improving productivity and performance by being more positive and focusing less on stress, negativity, and failures.

Health department managers and their teams in Wisconsin used quality improvement (QI) principles, processes, and tools to analyze root causes of identified challenges, and they created a focus at work-unit level to address indicators of employee engagement, including energy and vigor, engagement, and absorption. Each manager received monthly education on QI and "happiness advantage principles" and was assigned a QI coach; a short monthly all-staff "pulse" survey monitored improvements. Teams across the organization developed and led small projects to improve engagement that included activities to support getting to know one another better and stronger connectedness, supporting self-care breaks and adding walking breaks, creating exercise groups, increasing recognition and rewards, emphasizing kindness to others, making improvements to the physical space, coordinating workloads, and improving meetings.

Throughout the three-year implementation effort, the state collected data to monitor improvements and saw a significant increase in the key indicator "I recommend my organization as a good place to work," moving from 65% in 2017 to 74% in 2018. Today, the state continues to build on these efforts. Factors that were critical to the agency's success were highly engaged and visible leadership throughout the initiative, regular training and support for managers and staff, using QI processes to identify and pilot change projects, collecting and using data to monitor improvements, communicating regularly to share progress and successful approaches, and aligning efforts to support the agency's public health re-accreditation efforts.

Wisconsin's efforts produced marked improvements in staff morale and overall employee engagement. The agency continues to present both the foundational trauma-informed awareness training as well as the adapted *Happiness Advantage* training in all new-employee orientations. Institutionalizing these efforts is an important priority for the future, because it shows a commitment to creating a resilient workforce across administrations and can offer benefits to staff during periods of increased stress. The COVID-19 pandemic is a glaring example of an additional stressor that is affecting staff at public health agencies both personally and professionally and underscores the importance of efforts to support staff who may be struggling through agency connectedness and promotion of self-care.

What Managers Can Do

According to Gallup, managers account for 70% of the variance in employee engagement scores across business units.[12] The importance of managers in creating a culture that engages employees cannot be overstated. Given the significance of engagement and motivation on individual and organizational performance, managers should consider how they approach the following:

- Building psychological safety and trust. Leaders achieve this by demonstrating respect, being genuine and approachable, showing fairness and transparency in decision-making, being humble and admitting mistakes, acknowledging and overcoming their own biases, and seeing mistakes and failures as learning opportunities.
- Strengthening communication. Employees who believe their voices are heard are nearly five times more likely to feel empowered to perform their best work.[13] In 2021, PH WINS found that less than half of the workforce described communication between senior leadership and employees as good, suggesting room for improvement in this area.[14] Managers should ask staff about what matters to them, what meaning they find in their work, and how they feel connected to the larger purpose of the organization.
- Talking regularly with staff members about the meaning and purpose they see in their work and showing how their work aligns with the organizational mission.
- Crafting jobs or assigning new responsibilities based on staff members' values, strengths, and passions.
- Minimizing excessive or unnecessary rigidity. Managers need to consider what flexibilities may exist within the system: While there may be limits on what a manager can control, managers do have some discretion in how policies and procedures are implemented. Staff today want more work–life integration, so it is important to grant flexibility when possible, such as in scheduling work time. IHI describes this as pinpointing the "pebbles in our shoes."[11] This is about finding the processes, issues, and situations that get in the way of what matters at work.
- Assuring staff that they have some autonomy and choice in how they go about their work.
- Providing praise and recognition of individual and team performance and celebrating outcomes. Most employees feel

they do not receive enough praise or recognition. Rewards do not need to be monetary.

- Giving regular feedback and creating a culture of feedback throughout the agency. Feedback from peers can be just as meaningful, if not more so, than feedback from a supervisor. Feedback should be specific, timely, and actionable regardless of who gives it.
- Building camaraderie and teamwork. A study by Buckingham and Goodall found that employees are twice as likely to be engaged if they are doing most of their work in teams.
- Promoting positivity, a healthy work environment, wellness, and resiliency. Meditation, exercise, consciously performing acts of kindness, and making a daily list of the good things in your job, career, and life are simple ways to increase happiness.[11] Wisconsin's health department found that walking breaks and making small improvements to physical spaces were simple and effective changes that created a more positive and healthier work environment.
- Taking steps to demonstrate a commitment to diversity, equity, and inclusion. Managers should consider where unconscious biases may show up in hiring, performance reviews, and other day-to-day interactions. In addition to being authentic in building relationships with employees and working to ensure that all staff feel comfortable speaking openly, managers and leaders must support and advocate for inclusive and equitable organizational policies.

Summary

The public health workforce is passionate about, and dedicated to, its work. Managers and leaders can leverage this passion to help build employee motivation and engagement. While there are barriers in governmental systems that make extrinsic motivation challenging, leaders can create cultures that build upon intrinsic motivators to keep employees engaged. This chapter highlights some of the ways that governmental public health managers and leaders can increase employee engagement and unlock employee motivation by leveraging the important purpose and meaningful work of governmental public health; the chapter includes an example of this effort from the Wisconsin State Health Department. Even with the challenges posed by COVID-19, agencies can, and must, focus on employee engagement and help build employee resilience. Supervisors and managers, who have the most direct impact on employee motivation, are urged to use the tactics suggested here to embrace their roles in creating inclusive work environments that are engaging and satisfying for the very dedicated and diverse professionals with whom they work.

References

1. Robin Taylor Wilson, Catherine L. Troisi, and Tiffany L. Gary-Webb, "A Deficit of 250,000 Public Health Workers Is No Way to Fight Covid-19," *STAT News*, April 5, 2020, https://www.statnews.com/2020/04/05/defi cit-public-health-workers-no-way-to-fight-covid-19.
2. Rivka Liss-Levinson, "Update on Public Sector Employee Views on Finances and Employment Outlook Due to COVID-19: May vs. October 2020," January 2021, https://slge.org/assets/uploads/2021/01/jan2 021-slge-covid-report.pdf.
3. de Beaumont Foundation and Association of State and Territorial Health Officials (ASTHO), *Public Health Workforce Interests and Needs Survey: 2021 Findings*, https://www.debeaumont.org/findings/.
4. Josh Bersin, "Employee Retention Now a Big Issue: Why the Tide Has Turned," August 16, 2013, https://www.linkedin.com/pulse/2013081 6200159-131079-employee-retention-now-a-big-issue-why-the-tide-has-turned.
5. Peter Cappelli and Liat Eldor, "Where Measuring Engagement Goes Wrong," *Harvard Business Review* May (2019), https://hbr.org/2019/05/where-measuring-engagement-goes-wrong.
6. Marcus Buckingham and Ashley Goodall, "The Power of Hidden Teams," *Harvard Business Review* May (2019), https://hbr.org/2019/05/the-power-of-hidden-teams.
7. Jim Harter, "4 Factors Driving Record-High Employee Engagement in U.S.," *Gallup Workplace,* May 17, 2019, https://www.gallup.com/workpl ace/284180/factors-driving-record-high-employee-engagement.aspx.
8. Randall Beck and Jim Harter, "Managers Account for 70% of Variance in Employee Engagement" *Gallup Business Journal* (2021), https://news.gal lup.com/businessjournal/182792/managers-account-variance-emplo yee-engagement.aspx.

9. J. Richard Hackman and Greg R. Oldham, "Motivation through the Design of Work: Test of a Theory," *Organizational Behavior and Human Performance* 16, no. 2 (1976): 250–279, https://doi.org/10.1016/0030-5073(76)90016-7.

10. Jessica Perlo et al., *IHI Framework for Improving Joy in Work* (Cambridge, MA: Institute for Healthcare Improvement, 2017), https://www.ihi.org/resources/Pages/IHIWhitePapers/Framework-Improving-Joy-in-Work.aspx.

11. Shawn Achor, *The Happiness Advantage: The Seven Principles of Positive Psychology that Fuel Success and Performance at Work* (New York: Crown Publishing, 2010).

12. Gallup, *State of the American Workplace Report 2013*, https://www.gallup.com/file/services/176708/State%20of%20the%20American%20Workplace%20Report%202013.pdf.

13. Salesforce Research, *The Impact of Equality and Values Driven Business* (2017), https://www.salesforce.com/contents/impact-of-equality/.

14. de Beaumont Foundation and Association of State and Territorial Health Officials (ASTHO), *Public Health Workforce Interests and Needs Survey: 2017 Findings*, https://www.debeaumont.org/findings/.

11

STRATEGIC SKILLS IN FOCUS:
▶ *Data-Driven Decision-Making*

Using Data to Guide Public Health Action and Societal Change

CATHERINE C. SLEMP

Data-driven decision-making encompasses collecting, interpreting, and leveraging data to identify salient patterns, answer relevant questions, and make effective decisions. The insights generated during data analytics translate into tangible, real-world change and lead to informed action.[1] Using data to ground and guide decision-making, and ultimately to drive action and change, is both a critical skill and a central tenet of public health. Although large and formal data initiatives (mining big data for disaster response, collaborating on academic research, or using formal mathematical modeling, for example) may garner attention, equally or more significant are the less formal uses of data to guide internal public health agency processes and to shape externally facing policies and programs. Strategic leaders gather and use data to do such things as check assumptions, establish priorities, build a shared vision, evaluate programs, develop policy, engage stakeholders, or undertake advocacy. This chapter addresses these less formal but

Catherine C. Slemp, *Using Data to Guide Public Health Action and Societal Change* In: *Building Strategic Skills for Better Health: A Primer for Public Health Professionals*. Edited by: Michael R. Fraser and Brian C. Castrucci, Oxford University Press. © de Beaumont Foundation 2024. DOI: 10.1093/oso/9780197744604.003.0012 more common everyday uses of data by public health leaders. At its core, this leadership skill is about asking relevant questions—seeking to understand—and using the knowledge gained to improve health and well-being. It is aimed at targeting resources wisely, maximizing effectiveness, advancing equity, improving practice, defending actions, undertaking advocacy, engaging stakeholders, developing and supporting staff, and more.

Key Principles and Concepts in Using Data Strategically

In their description of Public Health 3.0, DeSalvo and colleagues note that "leaders serve as chief health strategists, partnering across multiple sectors and leveraging data and resources to address social, environmental, and economic conditions that affect health and health equity."[2] Doing so requires more than the technical or managerial aspects of ensuring that data are available and used. Strategically, there are several useful overarching concepts and principles. These are summarized in the following six principles.

Data in Their Traditional Form Typically Are Both Critically Important and Alone Insufficient for Sound Decision-making

While essential for setting priorities, planning work, communicating to stakeholders, or evaluating progress, data are just one key tool in decision-making. When using data to set priorities, for example, other factors to consider may include what is feasible, practical, politically acceptable, culturally relevant, or timely. Data on a particular health problem may identify an issue as being of utmost importance, but if the agency or organization is not in the position to address the issue, even with partners and collaborators, or if doing so will detract from other key initiatives, it may not be wise to prioritize the matter. In this situation, the data can instead become a strategic tool to advocate for improved resources, authority, re-examination of agency mission, or support of others in taking the lead on the issue at hand.

Choosing Which Data to Use Requires Being Both Selective and Flexible

Public health often is practiced in data-rich and information-poor environments. There may be more data than staff support to synthesize it, even with assistance from academic partners. The precise data desired may not be available or of perfect quality in the time needed, and the environment in which an agency is working on an issue may change over time. These factors speak to the importance of regularly assessing and strengthening agency informatics capability, proactively forming data-sharing and data-analysis partnerships, being deliberate in deciding what data to collect and use, and ensuring that evaluation is used for rapid improvement cycles. On any project and at key intervals, questions about selecting data may include:

- What indicators get at the crux of the issue and are actionable?
- What is readily available or able to be captured in the time needed?
- What is the quality of the data? How reliable, relevant, accurate, complete, and generalizable are the data?
- What data will best communicate to those engaged in decision-making or who are necessary to the success of an initiative (supervisors, policymakers, partners, media, program participants)?

Being Intentional about the Frame through Which Data Are Collected, Examined, and Communicated Can Affect How Others Engage (Assets- vs. Needs-based Approach)

Historically, public health has taken a needs-based approach to addressing problems. This has meant collecting data about where a problem is worst, discerning the risk factors associated with a disease or outcome, identifying gaps in the system, guiding service delivery, and so on. In writing grants, most authors focus on deficits in order to emphasize the need for resources to address an issue. Needs are real and important to acknowledge and understand.

Being intentional about gathering data on an individual or community's assets, strengths, hopes, and opportunities can prove a more effective way to engage others and to mobilize transformative and lasting change. With cross-sector support, individuals or communities often can capture where they are now, articulate a vision of where they want to go, and identify how to start the journey by building on identified internal assets potentially augmented with external resources. This is a more powerful, transformative, and sustainable way of advancing health than simply using facts or figures that reflect deficits followed by delivery of services. Similarly, presenting data and targets in the frame of the desired state (numbers of insured, numbers living in smoke-free housing) can be more engaging and visionary than presenting the same data using the negative frame (numbers of people who are not at a healthy weight, numbers of people who are not physically active).

Successful Leaders Will Avoid the Trap of Data Paralysis and Understand Its Causes

No data set is perfect or applicable to every situation, because public health takes on complex and adaptive societal problems (e.g., poverty, disease, disaster response, substance use, systemic inequities). Additional data, discussion, and study often help to get at root causes, engage new partners, and identify more creative and effective solutions. These are beneficial results, but agencies and groups can also find themselves stuck in the mode of ongoing study.

How much data or knowledge is sufficient? To answer this question, consider:

- Does the rigor and representativeness of the data available match the relevance and criticality of the problem?
- What is the cost of not moving forward with the data available?
- Is more or better data likely to change actions or impact plans and partnerships in the short or longer term?
- Is it more important to do something now and track progress with course corrections over time or to obtain a fuller understanding of the issue before tackling it?

- Are we getting lost in the volume or complexity of data or finding ourselves paralyzed by the lack thereof?

At times, consciously or subconsciously, the call for more data or analysis reflects other reasons for the hesitancy to act. These might include a politically uncomfortable situation, staff fatigue and burnout, need for additional time, distrust of partners, unrecognized biases, or differing value frameworks. Recognizing when the call for more data is masking these or other factors can help leaders address the underlying barriers (in themselves or in staff) in more effective and timely ways.

When Decisions Must Be Made before Data Are Either Sufficient Or Adequate, Intentional Measures to Reduce Risk Are Beneficial

Public health professionals and agencies highly value data and its intentional use, and rightfully so. Sometimes, however, necessary and/or sufficient data are not available when it is either politically or operationally essential to make a decision and move forward. This can be both discomforting and difficult. In disaster response, for instance, there often is no time to collect, or to wait for, important data. Deploying various approaches based on limited information can be both risky and life-saving.

Setting up systems for rapid cycle feedback or monitoring is critical. With COVID-19 outbreaks in nursing homes, for example, public health and healthcare professionals quickly found that some traditional influenza-like-illness laboratory testing and management approaches were inadequate for the SARS-CoV-2 virus. Alternative surveillance strategies and response measures emerged, some sooner than others, and experiential learning ensued. While the process was by no means perfect, risks were mitigated by ensuring strong communication among peers and with partners that created rapid peer learning and information-sharing communities. Peer learning was established among states through the Association of State and Territorial Health Officials (ASTHO), through state-based partnerships with long-term care associations, and with long-term care industry regional and national leadership.

Emergency situations also require strong public and political communication. This includes communicating the urgency of the situation, describing what is known and not known, articulating what is being done to learn more, and providing anticipatory information that actions and guidance are likely to change. Anticipatory messaging establishes change as a positive to expect, reflecting an agency's ability to identify and respond to new knowledge in a rapidly changing environment. This helps maintain cohesion and collaboration in times of uncertainty. Note that shifting the tolerance for risk can be as hard for public health staff, many of whom are accustomed to grounding their action in data, as it is for partners and the public. Leaders should be attuned to potential staff discomfort and needs in this regard.

The Approach Leaders Take to Data Becomes a Tangible Reflection of Their Own and Their Agency's Values and Priorities

The messaging, actions, priorities, and interests of public health leaders around data and its appropriate application actively help shape agency culture, credibility, transparency, partnerships, and public trust. The questions asked, the expectations set in job descriptions, the training and tools made available to staff, and the partnerships established all speak to an agency's value of grounding and guiding public health action and policy in data. In addition, the willingness of leaders to share and make data publicly available and interpretable (by partners, policymakers, and the public more broadly) can both support agency transparency and promote use of data in broader societal policymaking and practice. It also makes ongoing evaluation and continuous improvement more feasible, more effective, and an organizational norm.

Types of Data to Consider: Formal Versus Informal Data

Data for decision-making include traditional or formal epidemiologic data, both quantitative and qualitative, including data on demographics, health status, processes and outcomes, risk factors, geographic distribution, and healthcare access. These are the data collected through surveillance systems, public health or academic research, medical record abstractions, health information systems, and insurer data sets. They may include both quantitative and qualitative data from surveys, focus groups, social media reviews, key informant interviews, or community forums. Typically, data are systematically collected and analyzed. Health agencies collect much of the information themselves or engage other sources to collect it for them.

Beyond these traditional data types, it is useful to consider formal data on the environmental and cultural factors that influence policy and practice. Considerations include finding out what data are available that reflect political and societal will, community norms and values, or public opinion. Where possible, having agency capacity not only to identify but also to provide a basic assessment of the validity and applicability of these sources is helpful. The data can provide adjunct input to inform considerations like program or policy design, staffing, timing, communications, partner strategies, and use of resources.

Informal data, although somewhat less robust, are often readily accessible and potentially useful. Gathering such data can provide additional nuanced information, identify planning gaps, anticipate potential reactions, or garner ideas for new partners and resources. Relevant information can often be obtained through informally talking with, listening to, and bouncing ideas off community partners, stakeholders, trusted colleagues, or community influencers. Reviewing coverage of the issue at hand and current hot topics in local media (newspapers, radio, social media networks) helps leaders understand the context in which they're operating. This helps to gauge the enthusiasm with which a proposal may be met, identifies potential barriers or key opportunities, and can shape initiative timing, communication strategies, or the need to ensure that elected leadership is attuned to upcoming developments and the potential risks an action may bring.

Potential Data Sources

The opportunity to integrate data from various sources is growing, and new sources and tools arise regularly. Having a good working knowledge of publicly available sources, both internal and external to the organization, as well as data available through partners, is key. Each source has its own strengths, gaps, uses, and applicability. Driven by a focus on work at the community level, data are increasingly being made available at narrower jurisdictional levels (zip code, census tract, etc.). Many sites offer the ability to autogenerate county-level or smaller community profiles, augmenting the task of local community health assessments or examining vulnerability footprints across a jurisdiction. Sites that include not only health outcomes, access, and risk-factor data but also broader social determinants of health, civic engagement, or social cohesion data are a boon, and many sites combine data availability with evidence-based tools or road maps.

Nevertheless, challenges and room for growth in this area remain. The absence of nonproprietary tools for data, analytics, metrics, and other uses leaves actionable information out of reach for most localities.[3] Smaller and more rural areas often wrestle with the availability of locality-specific data, given data-collection limits and/or issues around small numbers and variability. It is important to consider the timeliness of the data if this is critical for the purpose at hand. Some sites now model estimates for locales (although often with wide confidence intervals). At times, primary sources may have more timely data sets or findings they are willing to share. When community-level information is insufficient, linking communities with academic partners, mobilizing communities themselves to support data collection, or augmenting the data available with community discussions aimed at uncovering and understanding deeper issues the data may not reflect can be beneficial. Partnerships are also useful when organizational capacity for data analytics or informatics is limited, an issue common to many governmental public health agencies. (See box 11.1 for examples of population health data sources.)

Data related to the operational functioning of public health agencies are valuable for assessing internal quality. Examples include data on agency personnel demographics, hiring processes, staff turnover, funding streams, and business processes. These data can be surprisingly hard to obtain because of data ownership issues across agencies,

---

BOX 11.1. EXAMPLES OF POPULATION HEALTH
DATA SOURCES

Examples of widely used population health data sources in the public domain include:

- County Health Rankings & Roadmaps: https://www.countyhealthranki ngs.org/
- CDC PLACES: https://www.cdc.gov/places/index.html
- Community Commons: https://www.communitycommons.org/collecti ons/Maps-and-Data
- AARP Livability Index: https://livabilityindex.aarp.org/
- CDC/ATSDR Social Vulnerability Index: https://www.atsdr.cdc.gov/pla ceandhealth/svi/index.html
- Opportunity Index: https://opportunityindex.org/
- U.S. Census: https://data.census.gov/cedsci/

Examples of agency-collected (or partner-collected) public health surveillance data include:

- National Notifiable Disease Surveillance System (NNDSS)
- Behavioral Risk Factor Surveillance System (BRFSS)
- Pregnancy Risk Assessment Monitoring System (PRAMS)
- Youth Risk Behavior Surveillance System (YRBSS)
- Cancer registry data
- Medicaid and other payer/cost data

---

legal issues, or dependence on the use of legacy or outdated systems. When such systems are updated, the ability to easily and accessibly produce meaningful and accurate information for action and quality improvement complementing their primary functional purpose should be given high priority. Leaders can project these needs and advocate for their inclusion.

Use of Data in Public Health

Data are vital both for guiding public health agency practices and programs and for establishing societal policies and environments essential to the health of individuals and communities. Six practical use cases for strategic ways to use public health and population data follow.

Agency Development and Quality Improvement

Applicable data and data-driven processes are critical to effective agency planning and quality-improvement efforts. Where is an agency now? Where does it need to go, given a current environmental scan and projected futures? What infrastructure is needed to get it there? How will the agency and those it is accountable to know that progress is being made?

Data are also critical to agency management. What may seem to be simple management questions (How long does it take to get funds out the door? How diverse or inclusive is our agency workforce? How well does it reflect populations experiencing disparities? How effective are we in our work?) are often complex and challenging to investigate and address. Yet these valuable data can inform, deepen conversations with staff, guide interventions and rapid improvement cycles, and track progress being made.

Data collection, evaluation, use, sharing, and transparency are integral to, and woven throughout, Public Health Accreditation Board Standards and Measures.[4] In 2019, it was estimated that 80% of the U.S. population was covered by an accredited state or local health department. However, experience related to COVID-19 as well as the challenges ahead—including climate change, chronic and infectious diseases, achieving health equity, and more holistically addressing substance use and mental health—suggest that continued development of the nation's public health infrastructure must occur. This includes ensuring that the skills, tools, people, and systems supporting robust data generation, analysis, and use are in place and sustainable. While not a replacement for investment and development, partnerships and collaborations clearly can augment efforts, especially in resource-strapped agencies.

Program Design and Evaluation

Technical, topic-specific advice about using data to plan, guide, and evaluate public health efforts is plentiful. Data can and should ground program design ranging from disease-specific interventions (HIV, TB, heart disease, etc.) to broader social determinants of health and health equity initiatives. Beyond the traditional uses of targeting resources and helping select effective interventions, data can be employed for ongoing program evolution and improvement. Given the natural human and organizational tendency to sustain the status quo, leaders should use data to help organizations, policymakers, and the public recognize the need for change. Programs and systems need ongoing, data-guided evaluation processes worked into their design for continuous quality-improvement purposes, impact measurement, accountability, and resource management.

In today's rapidly changing environments, data are also increasingly being used to guide communications campaigns. Here, data from focus groups, key informant interviews, or social media and network analyses can be useful. Such data were used, for example, to learn what terminology in a specific locale could help increase the credibility of health officials (referring to the "doctor in charge of flu for the state" rather than the "state health officer"), to craft language to more effectively engage people in services (publicizing "community immunization events" rather than "mass vaccination clinics"), and to identify specific messengers and language helpful for reaching various audiences as recommended by analysis of survey and focus group data.[5]

Driving Policy Change and Supporting Advocacy

Using data to inform and evaluate policy is crucial. Public health professionals often have the data, knowledge, communication skills, and access to policymakers that allow them to make the case for policy change at federal, state, and local levels. Shared effectively, data can be used to describe an issue, to estimate costs, to guide toward evidence-based solutions, and to project impact, including disparate or unintended consequences.

While policy ideally is grounded in, and informed by, data, it rarely is developed, passed, and implemented based on data alone. Shaping effective health policy is also supported by internally building or gaining access to the 5 *Essential Public Health Law Services*.[6] These include (1) access to evidence and expertise, (2) expertise in development of legal solutions, (3) collaborations that engage communities and build political will, (4) support for implementing, enforcing, and defending legal solutions, and (5) policy surveillance and evaluation.[3] Note that these activities begin and end with an emphasis on data guiding action.

In addition, using storytelling to reflect impact, finding experiential ways for policymakers to understand an issue or proposed solution, and engaging the power of community and/or partners to both shape solutions and to tell the story can be powerful and necessary adjuncts to using data in developing sound health policy.

Advancing Health Equity

In a just society, advancement of health equity and opportunity is at the core of population health leadership. Examining how public health collects, analyzes, interprets, communicates, and uses data will help uncover inequities and will identify policy, system, or environmental approaches to addressing them and to changing cultural norms more broadly. In working toward health equity, ask the following five questions:

1. *What data are collected?* Increasingly, but not yet universally, data are collected and explored by race, ethnicity, and language. Many other relevant factors are also associated with differences in opportunity for, or systemic barriers to, optimal health. Depending on the topic at hand and relevant to local context, these factors may include class, socioeconomic status, geographic locale, age, sex, gender identity, sexual orientation, disability, or mental health.

2. *Who collects, evaluates, interprets, and uses the data?* Engaging affected individuals and other stakeholders in each of these activities can both profoundly influence the quality of the data (both quantitative and qualitative) and help give voice to, and transfer leadership and power to, populations historically kept from such conversations by structural and systemic barriers.

3. *Who will have access to the data and in what form?* Regardless of who collects and analyzes data, data access in useful forms can strengthen the ability of marginalized or disenfranchised communities to engage in policy change and to regain agency in shaping their own future.

4. *What safe spaces are available or can be created for relevant stakeholders to collectively understand disparities, follow trends, identify and engage in solutions, or evaluate impact across sectors?* In their health strategist role, leaders can use data as one tool for connecting disparate entities across norms, values, and sectors, helping build the relationships, understanding, and trust needed to define and address systemic issues.

5. *Whose data are they to share and whose story is it to tell?* Considering issues of data ownership, confidentiality, privacy, respect, and ethics is important. This is especially, though not uniquely, true in using stories, narratives, photos, or art to share or communicate data. While public health leaders should, and do, champion health equity issues themselves, it is frequently either more appropriate or more powerful to support others in doing so by elevating the strengths, assets, visibility, and engagement of partners and affected community members.

Engaging Community and Related Stakeholders; Supporting Community-Led Change

Health is most effectively and equitably strengthened over the long term when work is done by or with a community, not to or for them. The way public health professionals obtain, handle, and use data is paramount in supporting and facilitating this. In his summary of methods and approaches to understanding behavior and societal change, Avis writes, "Information alone is insufficient to support behavior change. Influencing healthy behaviors and creating a supportive social environment in a variety of contexts requires stimulation of learning and participation."[7] The acts of collecting, analyzing, interpreting, and using data can be powerful tools for building trust with communities, for engaging and mobilizing others, and for supporting community-led change. These processes can be used as collective areas of involvement, learning, and discovery.

How one approaches data with a community or community coalition can be pivotal. Are data being used to ask questions and guide collective efforts or to give answers and justify programs? With the former, data can help open a conversation, clarify an issue, identify local priorities, or build collaboration and trust. To advance toward community-led change, consider the following:

- Do the data resonate with community members? Why or why not?
- What deeper issues might be reflected?
- Who else cares or might have insights?
- What community and partner assets and gifts are relevant and available?
- What are the next steps forward?

In an environment of trust, such questions can be conversations of invitation or can spark partnership, collaboration, or coalition development. They can also be the start of community-led movements. In environments of distrust, this inquiry can instigate rebuilding of the trust needed to move forward.

For areas that the community has prioritized, engaging localities in, and equipping them for, their own data collection, interpretation, and use can be remarkably effective. This may take the form of tools, such as photovoice participatory research, youth-led research projects, or formal community-led research. While at times labor-intensive, such efforts can help mobilize and build powerful, effective, and more sustainable policy and environmental change. Among the tools that support use of data by coalitions and community-led initiatives are those specifically attuned to issues of equity, such as the California Opioid Prevention Network's (COPN) *Guide to Measurement*[8] and Chicago Beyond's *Why Am I Always Being Researched?*[9] Besides providing interactive tools to help coalitions leverage data to guide program and policy decisions, target health inequities, and communicate with core audiences, the COPN tool also links to resources for evaluating coalition and collaboration effectiveness. The Chicago Beyond tool reckons with the issue of unintended bias in community research and works to level the playing field. As noted in this guide, "If evidence matters, we must care how it gets made."[9]

Building Community Trust, Establishing Relevance, and Serving as a Public Asset

How an agency collects, frames, and makes data readily available to others can establish the agency as a public asset, build agency relevance, and advance public trust. Assess the following about an agency's relationship with its community:

- To what extent does the agency speak to, and live out, the value of using quality data to shape programs or policy?
- Does it make data readily available in timely and understandable formats to the public, policymakers, and the media? Is this done as a user-driven service (many agencies now utilize dashboards to make common data readily available to all) or must the data be requested? How easy is the process?
- Are data handled appropriately with regard to privacy and confidentiality? Are data released with a reasonable balancing of the need for both agency transparency and service and maintenance of confidentiality, where appropriate?
- How openly and transparently are data errors handled and communicated?

The infrastructure behind making good-quality and timely data widely available is complex and includes putting in place strong data collection mechanisms and partnerships; tools that support timely and accurate data collection, evaluation, and visualization; personnel skilled in, and available for, both informatics and quality improvement; and systems—policies, processes, and legal authorities—for sharing or exchanging data with others. The push for almost instantaneous, real-time, accurate data related to COVID-19 severely stretched and exceeded the capabilities of many health agencies, revealing the opportunity to drive public health innovations and technology advances forward. Supporting public understanding of data collection and advancing data literacy are related goals.

Understanding Human Decision-making Informs How Data Are Used

System factors (ease of access, cost, historical context, social environment, etc.) logically feed into human decision-making. In addition, public health work is frequently undertaken in a culture and environment of information overload, social media, cultural upheaval, and political polarization. Helpful in moving data to action is a basic understanding of human decision-making and social psychology. These suggest that for reasons related to evolution and to efficiency, human decision-making primarily uses the "intuitive brain," with only a small percentage of decisions (~10%) engaging the "rational brain."[10] Soosalu et al. write about the decision-making components of "head (rational), heart (emotional), and gut (intuitive)."[11]

The fact that more than rationality is at play does not mean that decisions made are rarely good or reasonable, but that human decisions and judgment are not as rational, data-driven, or straightforward as public health professionals might think. Other sociopsychological factors (for example, the parallel desires to both be unique and to belong to the group, cultural norms and values, confirmation bias, or a desire for quick fixes to complex truths) have an effect as well. Understanding the complexity of human decision-making helps public health leaders more effectively shape their approach to guiding policy.

Such understanding can help leaders avoid, for example, the pitfall of basing policy communications on data alone (speaking solely to the rational brain), recognizing that doing so may at best be insufficient and at worst lead to blatant distrust and dissent. Tapping into empathy (storytelling, visual representations) and relationships (using trusted messengers, building pre-existing relationships, identifying commonalities) and communicating data and information in ways that speak to an audience's or community's values and frameworks are all important tools in applying the information data provides. Leaders with an understanding of moral foundation theory, as described in the National Network of Public Health Law's article "Becoming Better Messengers"[10] and leaders who understand the science of framing, for example using the FrameWorks Institute's "Framing 101" resources[12] will be more effective at applying data to action, policy, and change.

From Theory to Practice: Everyday Ways to Strengthen the Use of Data in Advancing Health and Well-being

Public health leadership skills in wisely, adeptly, and ethically using data to ground policy, to guide organizational development, to engage others, to drive social change, or to establish a culture that values and uses data effectively are vital to our collective efforts to advance the health of individuals and populations. Leaders can embody and practice these skills in a variety of ways. They can help ensure that the data their agency collects or utilizes and the processes around which it is handled and shared intentionally embody values of equity, partnership, transparency, and mutual accountability.

In developing programs and policies, leaders can engage communities and other stakeholders in ways that honor an affected population's ability to collect, interpret, and tell its own story or shape its own solutions using data. They can commit resources to ensure that staff have the tools and skills needed to ground decisions in data and to communicate that data effectively to varied audiences. Leaders can ask reflective questions that use and value data both in internal discussions and in work with partners. They can model both being adept at understanding data and its limitations and humble in listening to communities and partners about what may be behind observed trends or what may be most effective in addressing them. These are skills and practices that warrant intentionality and continuous honing through experience, practice, mentoring, or reflective learning in dialogue with cross-sector peers.

Data-driven decision-making skills help us navigate systems and advance change. These skills must be combined with, and used to support and complement, other strategic leadership skills in public health. It is in applying these skills together that we most effectively and meaningfully shape the systems, policies, and environments—or even create and advance entire movements—that allow individuals, families, and communities to thrive, grow, and change.

References
1. Moriah Gendelman, Samantha Cinnick, and Grace Castillo, *Adapting and Aligning Public Health Strategic Skills*, de Beaumont Foundation,

March 2020, https://debeaumont.org/wp-content/uploads/2021/04/Adapting-and-Aligning-Public-Health-Strategic-Skills.pdf.

2. Karen B. DeSalvo et al., "Public Health 3.0: A Call to Action for Public Health to Meet the Challenges of the 21st Century," *Preventing Chronic Disease* 17 (2017), https://www.cdc.gov/pcd/issues/2017/17_0017.htm.

3. *Standards and Measures for Initial Accreditation*, Public Health Accreditation Board, December 2013, https://phaboard.org/standards-and-measures-for-initial-accreditation/.

4. *Changing the COVID Conversation*, de Beaumont Foundation, https://deb eaumont.org/changing-the-covid-conversation/.

5. Colleen Barbero et al., "7 Things You Should Know about Legal Epidemiology," *Public Health Management and Practice Direct*, February 11, 2020, https://jphmpdirect.com/2020/02/11/seven-things-you-sho uld-know-about-legal-epidemiology/.

6. Scott Burris et al., "Better Health Faster: The 5 Essential Public Health Law Services," *Public Health Reports* 131, no. 6 (2016): 747–753, https://pubmed.ncbi.nlm.nih.gov/28123219/.

7. William Robert Avis, *Methods and Approaches to Understanding Behaviour Change*, (Birmingham, UK: GSDRC, University of Birmingham, 2016), https://gsdrc.org/publications/methods-and-approaches-to-understand ing-behaviour-change.

8. California Opioid Prevention Network (COPN), *Measurement Guide*, 2021, https://nopn.org/resources/copn-measurement-guide.

9. *Why Am I Always Being Researched? A Guidebook for Community Organizations, Researchers, and Funders to Help Us Get from Insufficient Understanding to More Authentic Truth*, Chicago Beyond, 2018, https://chicagobeyond.org/researchequity.

10. "Becoming Better Messengers," The Network for Public Health Law, https://www.networkforphl.org/resources/topics/trainings/becoming-better-messengers.

11. Grant Soosalu, Suzanne Henwood, and Arun Deo, "Head, Heart, and Gut in Decision-making: Development of a Multiple Brain Preference Questionnaire," *Sage Open* 9, no. 1 (2019), https://journals.sagepub.com/doi/full/10.1177/2158244019837439.

12. "Framing 101," The FrameWorks Institute, https://www.frameworksin stitute.org/tools-and-resources/framing-101.

Strategic Resource Management

EDWARD M. CAHILL

COVID-19 HAS DEMONSTRATED THE URGENT need for agencies to address procurement challenges and hiring barriers and to engage subject matter experts and community partners more efficiently through innovative fiscal partnerships and personnel arrangements. Dealing with issues like COVID-19, measles, West Nile, Zika, the opioid crisis, environmental hazards, and drug-resistant diseases, such as MRSA and staph infections, along with routine public health duties, strains existing resources and can impede typical operations when appropriate personnel and policies are not in place to quickly pivot to new priorities and agency functions.

Two areas of focus for public health professionals interested in improving business operations are resource acquisition and utilization of existing resources. As this chapter describes, when these two areas are cultivated by program staff, strategic resource usage will be enhanced, and public health programs will be better able to cope with the demands they face. Staff also will be better able to respond to ever-increasing pressures for accountability from their supervisors, the public, and elected officials.

Edward M. Cahill, *Strategic Resource Management* In: *Building Strategic Skills for Better Health: A Primer for Public Health Professionals*. Edited by: Michael R. Fraser and Brian C. Castrucci, Oxford University Press.
© de Beaumont Foundation 2024. DOI: 10.1093/oso/9780197744604.003.0013

Resource Acquisition

One of the most important functions of an organization's management is to ensure that agency programs have sufficient resources to perform project tasks. Everything that an agency does requires funding. In the public sector, obtaining funding requires budgeting. Hiring staff, promoting staff, buying supplies and equipment, and issuing contracts all require funds. People with a solid knowledge of the principles of budgeting and finance know the ins and outs of acquiring resources for their programs, and that knowledge in turn allows each program to provide optimal services to its clients. Similarly, in the public sector, budgeting and financial acumen are required for effective stewardship of agency resources.

Periodically, agencies submit budget requests to elected officials. A compelling justification is essential to ensure approval of the budget request, which must provide all the essential information needed for reviewers to completely understand the initiative. The request must also be clear and concise. Too often, program staff provide incomplete information with the assumption that everyone understands the need and is familiar with the issues being addressed. The request could be critical, but individuals outside an immediate program area cannot be expected to be as familiar with an issue as program staff are. Unless an initiative is thoroughly explained, the likelihood of receiving funding is greatly reduced.

For example, program staff dealing with a serious environmental contamination issue submitted a request for a $1 million mass spectrometer but included no explanation of why the instrument was necessary to analyze soil samples. In this case, because of the serious nature of the issue, clarification was requested and the funding was provided. However, because of the lack of justification in the initial request, the need for this vital equipment was nearly overlooked by the policymakers making budgetary decisions for the agency.

Budget requests that include statistics—data, facts, and figures—are more easily justified and compelling than requests that do not. When a program can develop units of workload or unit costs, the justification for increased funding is enhanced. In the case of a local health department doing sanitary inspections of restaurants, an inspector on average can complete 100 restaurant inspections a year. If there are 2,000 restaurants required to be inspected once every two years, then 10 inspectors are needed to handle the workload (1,000 restaurants to be inspected every year divided by 100 inspections per employee equals 10 inspectors). If increasing the inspection rate from once every two years to once annually is proposed to combat outbreaks of food-borne illness, then the need for an additional 10 inspectors can be easily shown (2,000 annual restaurant inspections divided by 100 inspections per employee equals 20 inspectors to handle the increased workload). Spelling out the need in detail provides better support for the initiative than merely asking for more inspectors.

Another tactic that increases the chances for approval of a budget request is including information on the return on investment (ROI). When preparing requests for new resources, the justification and hence the likelihood of approval improve when the request shows that the initiative will provide benefits that exceed the cost. A cost–benefit analysis of a nutrition program has shown that every dollar spent on that program, which provides nutritious food for low-income individuals, results in five times the savings in future medical costs. Thus, the cost of the program can be categorized as an investment and not just as an expenditure. In particular, the investment will provide substantial future cost savings for publicly funded programs like Medicaid.

While the obvious reason for the program is to improve the health of participants, the added benefit of future cost savings makes the program more attractive to decision makers. Not all necessary and desirable expenditures can be reduced to a dollars-and-cents analysis, but those that can, and that show a positive ROI, will be better supported in the decision-making process.

Identifying alternative revenue sources is another way to elicit support for additional resources. At the state and local levels, most expenditures are supported by tax dollars, through property taxes, sales taxes, or income taxes. Public aversion to taxes is well known, and elected officials endeavor to keep taxes low and under control. If a proposed budget initiative lends itself to self-financing either in whole or in part, that can improve its chances for approval. Voluntary fees for desirable public health activities, fines for illegal or egregious activities (such as the sale of alcohol or tobacco to underage individuals), donations from benefactors, and grants from the federal government and philanthropic organizations are all possible alternative sources of funds but can also become targets of industry advocates who may oppose them. Any source of funds that mitigates the use of tax dollars to support new resources improves the chances for increased funding.

There is often a tendency to "pad" budget requests by inflating the actual amount needed to accomplish an initiative. This may take the form of asking for more staff than are needed or increasing the proposed budget for supplies and equipment; it might involve exaggerating the need to deal with the problem. All budget requests are reviewed by staff who are professionals in the funding process. If they repeatedly see requests from a particular program or individual that are for amounts above reasonable levels, they bear that in mind when making funding recommendations. At times, decision makers will not have all the information they need to justify approving a request. In that case, the reputation of the requester may determine the success of the request. If the requester is regarded as knowledgeable, truthful, and reasonable, and can be relied upon to provide an honest justification for the request and its level of funding, the decision maker is more likely to approve the request. However, if the requester is known as someone who consistently inflates the need for resources, the decision maker may balk at a favorable recommendation. Attempts to gain a one-time advantage by being less than forthright typically cause future pitfalls.

Utilization of Existing Resources

In the current fiscal environment, obtaining new resources for programs is difficult at best; programs need to get the most from existing resources to meet the demands they face. Flexibility is key, but often in the public sector, well-intentioned rules and regulations, as well as traditional practices, instill a spirit of rigidity into operations. Program staff need to develop practices that allow better deployment of existing resources. The most important resource any organization has is its employees—capable, motivated, and dedicated staff are required for a program to succeed. Fortunately, most public health programs are staffed by such people, because the sector attracts those who are ready, willing, and able to do what it takes to help individuals and society. But dynamics like antiquated civil service rules, categorical funding restrictions, and organizational territorial concerns can restrict the best use of employees.

One constraint on effective use of employees is overly specific civil service titles and job categories that limit the type of work employees can perform. While civil service is designed to be a merit system and to ensure that public programs get the best employees for their positions, the approach can provide unintentional obstacles for managers and staff. The proliferation of unique job titles in the effort to enumerate the precise specifications required for each position is often unnecessary and limits the employee to a narrow area of work. Managers are limited in which program areas the position can be deployed to, and the employee is limited in the work to which he or she can officially be assigned.

For example, in disease investigations, the principles of contact tracing are the same regardless of the disease being investigated. There is no need to develop separate civil service job titles, such as Sexually Transmitted Disease (STD) Investigator and Tuberculosis Investigator, in which each has different qualifications and the incumbent is relegated to working solely on that specific disease. Both programs would be better off with a common job title that allows interchange of staff as needed. That way, additional personnel resources can be marshaled quickly as conditions require, the pool of employees eligible to work on assignments is larger, and management has more personnel options.

Another limit on flexibility of personnel assignments is the categorical nature of funding. Staff in public health programs are usually paid from multiple funding sources. Specific sources of monies include categorical federal grants and special revenue accounts from sources like fees and fines associated with a particular program. The funding source provides the money for a special purpose and typically restricts expenditures from those funds to the designated purpose.

Thus, positions on different fund sources in the same title and in the same agency may not be able to work interchangeably on the same program. Investigators funded on a federal categorical STD grant cannot work on an immunization investigation if the STD grant is being charged for the salary of the investigators doing the immunization work. Essentially, if a grant is paying for an expenditure, the effort behind that expenditure must be for the same purpose as the specific grant. While this restriction may be waived by funders during emergencies, such as in the COVID-19 response, in typical operations it creates barriers to staff sharing and surge capacity when needed.

While understandable, making the efforts exclusive to each fund source can result in the inability to use resources most efficiently. Programs can get around exclusivity of funding by developing a method to properly charge to a fund source not only the salary of employees but also the activity and effort of the employees. In other words, an employee can work in areas other than those of a designated fund source and still avoid the misuse of funds and audit exceptions so long as the time, effort, and corresponding dollar amounts of the person's salary are charged to appropriate fund sources. A simple way to do this would be to have each employee certify the programs worked on during each pay period and the amount of time devoted to each one. The proportional amount of salary can then be moved to each fund source.

Periodic assessments utilizing data gathered in fiscal operations can provide a solid basis to help program decisions on deployment of available resources. Is the program using its resources in the best way? Where can improvements be made? Is the program operating effectively and efficiently? Underutilized or inappropriately used resources should be redeployed to more productive uses.

Consider a program that provides funds to local clinics for free medical exams in low-income populations. A simple analysis of the program would divide the amount of funding provided to each clinic by the number of medical exams it performed, to obtain the average cost of an examination at each clinic. If there are significant differences in the average costs, the program should ask why. Some of the differences could easily be explained as cost-of-living differences between urban and rural areas, but other differences might not be as obvious. Some clinics may have richer staffing patterns than others but deliver the same number of exams with the same quality. In cases where higher-than-ordinary costs are deemed unnecessary, those higher expenditures can be reduced to bring the average cost of an exam in line with the cost at most clinics. In cases where the average cost is significantly below the average cost of the group, specific reasons should be ascertained, and the efficiencies communicated to other clinics as best practices. In both cases, savings resulting from the analysis can be redeployed to provide more medical exams, thereby enhancing the program's overall effectiveness.

Program managers also can use comparative funding data to analyze costs and results in different agencies or jurisdictions. Just because a program has more resources or costs than another program does not mean that its results will be better. Many times, after comparing costs of comparable programs in different agencies or jurisdictions, managers find that the cost of added resources results in no significant difference in outcomes. A good example is a program that requires annual on-site inspections of all food service establishments. That program costs three times as much to operate as another program in a separate jurisdiction that requires an on-site inspection only once every three years. If there is no difference in the incidence of food-borne disease outbreaks between the two programs, the costlier program could consider changing its inspection schedule and redeploying the savings into a more productive area.

Ongoing monitoring of a program's expenditures during the year by program staff to maximize resources cannot be overemphasized. Program staff may view budgeting and fiscal activities only as ways to avoid overspending. The reality is that proper fiscal oversight also avoids underspending of funds. If a public health program is provided an appropriation and it is not spent, it means that services needed by the public are not being provided at the level the appropriating body intended. All programs can have delays in making planned expenditures, and underspending can result from issues like delays in hiring qualified staff and in issuing timely contracts. If program staff are aware of the accruing under-expenditures, those savings can be redeployed to other essential areas.

A jaded interpretation of the expression "use it or lose it" would imply a need to spend all available funding during a budget year whether needed or not. But in public health, the need for additional funds is so great that any found savings from underspending should always be put to an essential use; allowing any funds to go unused is a serious mistake. An effective monitoring system can easily be set up to avoid underspending: programs should budget their appropriated funds by object of expense (salaries, supplies, equipment, travel, contracts, etc.) and should estimate monthly expenditures that will occur in each category. A monthly comparison of actual expenditures to planned expenditures allows adjustments to be made over the remaining months of the year. These adjustments allow for maximum use of available resources by reducing or eliminating underspending.

Another way staff can optimize the use of program resources is through networking. Although networking is defined as the exchange of information among people with a common profession or special interest, it should be much more than that. It needs to be about developing and sustaining long-term relationships. Networking is important in all aspects of professional life, not least of which is resource management. During a temporary shutdown of the federal government a few years ago, several public health program staff in different states held impromptu conference calls to discuss the situation and how programs in each state were handling potential funding delays. The exchange of information aided several localities in adopting measures that mitigated the delay of federal funds during the shutdown. Contacts among program staff allowed information-sharing and adoption of best practices among participants. National associations, such as the Association of State and Territorial Health Officials, play a role in promoting such networking opportunities and in supporting peer groups doing similar work in different states.

Savvy program staff also cultivate contacts within their own agencies, particularly in the agency fiscal office. Governmental fiscal systems are often arcane and complex to navigate, and staff in fiscal offices are the experts in financial matters. They can provide the advice and assistance programs needed both to acquire and to use resources effectively. Many laws, rules, and regulations have been instituted in the public sector to minimize misuse of funds and to promote public objectives, such as nondiscrimination in awarding contracts and purchasing goods and services. Unless carefully navigated, these administrative requirements can be frustrating and difficult, especially for staff unfamiliar with the process. Agency fiscal staff know best how to tackle complex administrative requirements: what needs to happen, when it needs to happen, and how to quickly get external approvals. This guidance helps ensure effective and efficient delivery of services and reduces complications for program staff.

Summary

Staff in public health programs can increase the health outcomes of their programs by cultivating the strategic skills involved in budgeting and fiscal management. Rather than having these areas be seen as a necessary chore, they should be regarded as an opportunity to maximize the resources needed to accomplish program objectives. Two principles to consider are resource acquisition and utilization of current existing resources.

Justice, Equity, Diversity, and Inclusion in Public Health

Leveraging the Power of Diverse Teams to Optimize the Public's Health

MICHAEL R. FRASER

AS THE COUNTRY'S POPULATION BECOMES increasingly diverse,[1] public health agencies are adapting to meet the challenges and opportunities the changing demographics present to contemporary public health practice. To build trust and legitimacy in its work, governmental public health must ensure that the teams of practitioners serving the communities reflect the diversity of their populations. The recent experience of planning for, and distributing, COVID-19 vaccines demonstrates just how important this is: public health and healthcare leaders from different backgrounds and experiences delivered tailored messages to specific racial and ethnic groups that addressed specific historic or cultural concerns about vaccine safety and helped grow confidence in the public health system.[2,3]

This chapter summarizes the benefits and opportunities of an intentional focus on recruiting and retaining diverse teams for

Michael R. Fraser, *Justice, Equity, Diversity, and Inclusion in Public Health* In: *Building Strategic Skills for Better Health: A Primer for Public Health Professionals.* Edited by: Michael R. Fraser and Brian C. Castrucci, Oxford University Press. © de Beaumont Foundation 2024. DOI: 10.1093/oso/9780197744604.003.0014 governmental public health agencies. Employing a diverse workforce does not guarantee, however, that agency programs and services will become more effective. Managers and leaders need to create the conditions that allow diverse teams to thrive in their organizations and, by extension, to improve the health of their communities.

Diversity in Today's Public Health Workforce

National data from the 2021 Public Health Workforce Interests and Needs (PH WINS) survey suggest that the public health workforce at the state, territorial, and local levels mostly mirrors the racial and ethnic diversity of the nation (see table 13.1). More research is needed to describe the racial and ethnic composition of the workforce in each state or local jurisdiction and to assess how representative the national workforce is of some racial and ethnic groups, including Native American and Alaska Natives, and Native Hawaiian and other Pacific Islanders.[4] Data from the 2021 PH WINS show that 66% of the executive workforce in governmental public health agencies is female and 79% of the entire workforce is female. It follows that for men, a higher percentage hold public health leadership positions than they represent in the workforce overall.[4,5]

Table 13.1. Race, Ethnicity, and Gender Characteristics of State, Territorial, and Select Local Public Health Agency Workforces Compared to U.S. Population

	PH WINS* (2021)	U.S. Population (2021)
Race and Ethnicity		
White, non-Hispanic	54%	59%
Black, non-Hispanic	15%	14%
Hispanic or Latino	18%	19%
Asian	7%	6%
Two or more races	4%	3%
Gender		
Female	79%	51%
Male	20%	49%
Nonbinary/Other	2%	Not collected

Source: PH WINS 2021 survey and U.S. Census Bureau, "Quick Facts: People" available from https://www.census.gov/quickfacts/fact/table/US/PST045219. Totals do not add to 100% due to rounding error. *Note: PH WINS included local health departments and city health agencies with 25 or more staff members; other local health agencies are not included in the data.

Many studies in the business administration, management, and organizational development literature demonstrate how and why diversity and inclusion, especially work by diverse and inclusive teams, generate improved results for corporations and large firms, but little of this work has been applied to governmental organizations and nonprofit entities. Diversity and inclusion have been combined and prioritized as a critical strategic skill for public health agencies,[6] and human resource leaders and workforce planners in all levels of government are working to add diversity to the overall governmental workforce.

Broad attention to, and interest in, governmental diversity and inclusion are apparent in recent research by the Center for State and Local Government Excellence (SLGE), which highlighted diversity and inclusion as a significant trend to watch in 2021 and beyond, saying, "as public sector employers work to attract and retain a talented workforce of the future, they will look to ensure that their workforce is diverse, inclusive, and more reflective of the populations they serve."[7] A 2020 SLGE stakeholders meeting identified diversity and inclusion as vital to future governmental organizations and called on governmental leaders to create and maintain workplace cultures that support diversity and equity, to recruit and retain diverse employees, and to create a workplace culture that "welcomes their contributions, provides them with peer networks or affinity groups that support them, and training on topics [like] implicit bias to ensure that policies, procedures, or past practices do not create roadblocks to retention and career development."[8] These trends reflect the growing diversity of the population served by all levels of government, and the need to have a workforce that mirrors the diversity of racial, ethnic, religious, national origin, and other characteristics of the jurisdictions they serve. Practitioners from diverse backgrounds will support and assist community members in navigating government services and programs efficiently and effectively.

When considering workforce diversity and workplace inclusion, racial and ethnic diversity and the representation of different groups in a public health agency's workforce usually come to mind first. Research on management and organizational development suggests that organizations with a racially and ethnically diverse workforce are more creative and innovative and produce increased value for stakeholders over more homogeneous organizations. Studies on team performance and organizational effectiveness suggest that in addition to racial and ethnic identities, diversity and inclusion efforts should embrace identities like age, gender, sexual identity, religion, professional specialty, languages spoken, physical abilities, and others as an organization looks to bring varied experience and perspectives to its work and to produce better results for its stakeholders or "customers."

When the findings from corporate diversity efforts are applied to public health agencies, they reveal that a diverse and inclusive workplace culture creates several internal and external benefits. Externally, having staff who reflect the diverse populations in a jurisdiction may allow an organization to more easily develop trust with various communities and to be seen as a legitimate partner in community-based health promotion and disease prevention activities. The experience of community health workers is instructive: community health workers, such as *promotores de salud* (lay health workers), help individuals navigate the healthcare and public health system, develop trust with community members, and establish the enduring links needed to improve and sustain health over time.[9] Internally, bringing diverse staff together on public health teams allows for greater creativity and more successful outcomes for an agency because the lived experience of community members is reflected on the team and is included in program and policy development and implementation. When managed well, team diversity can lead to better-informed and more culturally responsive public health efforts.

The way an organization supports and manages diverse teams of public health professionals at the small functional level (work teams, units, branches, bureaus, divisions, and so on) is also critical to successfully accomplishing agency work in communities. At its core, public health is a "team sport." That is, the work of successful public health practice involves working with others on a team to achieve shared goals—little in public health can be done alone. Instead, public health work is performed by groups comprising various professionals in an agency who work together toward a common goal and serve a specialized function. Managing these diverse teams to tap into their collective expertise and maximize their contribution to the organization is a crucial role for leaders who desire to optimize agency performance and to generate optimal health in their communities.

Leveraging Diversity to Optimize the Public's Health

Contemporary public health practice involves agency staff serving on committees, work groups, task forces, and other groups to accomplish specific goals or tasks. However, there is a difference between a group and a team: a high-performing team is a specific kind of group, not an ad hoc collection of agency staff.[10] Like other work groups, teams share a unity of purpose and accountability for achieving a shared goal; they also bring a balance of requisite skills, abilities, and knowledge to their work that differentiates them from other groups. As Katzenbach and Smith write in the best-selling *The Wisdom of Teams*, "[A] team is a small number of people with complementary skills who are committed to a common purpose, performance goals, and approach for which they hold themselves mutually accountable."[11]

The business case for building and supporting diverse teams is well established in the literature on management and organizational behavior. As an example, a study of investment fund managers who worked on diverse teams with complementary skill sets found that the teams generated a significantly higher rate of return on investments that the team selected collectively.[12] In another study, global management consulting firm McKinsey found that, of 366 public companies, those in the top quartile for racial and ethnic diversity were 30% more likely to have financial returns above their respective national industry medians.[13] Companies in the bottom quartile for gender and for ethnicity and race were statistically less likely to achieve above-average financial returns than the average companies in the data set, indicating not just average, but lagging, performance.[13]

Primarily, diverse teams do better than nondiverse teams by intentionally focusing on bringing the team's perspectives, viewpoints, and experiences to its shared work.[14] This focus, along with commitment to the same goals and shared accountability for outcomes, leads to improved performance.[11] For example, efforts to increase vaccination among vaccine-hesitant populations have benefited from agency planning that includes members of those communities who are able to inform the development of messaging that resonates with different audiences, including those in different racial and ethnic groups. Similarly, efforts to end the HIV epidemic have supported public health agencies that form work teams that include members from communities who have been marginalized by discrimination and racism, such as transgender individuals and young Black men. With varied and diverse perspectives at the planning table, work on a variety of issues, from COVID-19 to HIV/AIDS, will be better informed by the experiences of those most adversely impacted.

Several researchers have investigated how diverse teams do better than nondiverse teams. Rock and Grant suggest that diverse teams are "smarter" because heterogeneous teams may be more aware of their own biases than homogeneous teams and may be more likely to re-examine something than a homogeneous group.[15] Members of diverse teams bring multiple perspectives to a shared task, which allows the group to consider alternative solutions for the problem at hand; on a diverse team, no single individual possesses the full range of knowledge or expertise needed to obtain a shared goal, and the collective wisdom of the group is tapped for relevant ideas and solutions.[14,16]

In addition, if members of a team are considering decisions about a community or group of which they are a part, the decisions reached may be more culturally relevant and better informed because they are based on shared, lived experience with members of that group. Diverse and inclusive teams also have an impact on organizational retention. When employees are engaged on diverse and inclusive teams, they are more likely to stay at an organization, because they are seen as valued members of a team and are more likely to be engaged in their work. This is especially true for millennials, who value diversity and look for inclusive workplaces to which they can contribute.[17]

Of course, the benefits of diverse teams cannot be realized solely by recruiting and retaining a diverse workforce. Diversity must be managed, and inclusion of various perspectives must be promoted and encouraged as part of an organization's workplace culture.[18] Katzenbach and Smith[10] explain supporting effective team performance as a discipline, which includes:

1. Creating a meaningful common purpose that the team helps to shape
2. Developing specific performance goals that flow from the common purpose
3. Ensuring that the team has the right mix of complementary skills
4. Reaching agreement and strong commitment about how the work gets done
5. Establishing mutual accountability

An organization supports its workforce by recruiting, hiring, and promoting employees of different racial, ethnic, gender, religious, and other identities. Efforts to support diverse work teams will fail if commensurate attention is not placed on eliminating systemic barriers to success for all employees. This includes antiracism efforts and leader commitments to supporting racial healing and transformation within an organization itself.[19] This work emphasizes the importance of what all employees bring to their shared workplace and seeks to dispel historic and systemic biases that promote hierarchies of human value based on race or national origin. To truly realize the benefits of diversity, leaders must create, manage, and nurture organizational cultures that support inclusion of different perspectives and experiences in organizational work and at the same time systematically confront racist, sexist, or other discriminatory or biased policies that have explicitly or implicitly perpetuated inequities. This means making the moral case for diversity and inclusion, not just the business case.

Diversity and Inclusion: From Business Case to Moral Case

In their article "Getting Serious About Diversity: Enough Already with the Business Case,"[20] Robin Ely and David Thomas—business school professors who were among the first to illustrate the importance of racial and gender diversity to organizational performance[21]—argue that organizations have a moral imperative, not solely a business imperative, to support efforts toward diversity and inclusion. Especially in research published following the nationwide protests of George Floyd's murder in May 2020, several authors have written that beyond recruiting and retaining employees of different racial and ethnic identities,[22,23] leaders need to grasp how their organizations perpetuate systemic oppression and discrimination and then work to dismantle racist, sexist, or other discriminatory policies or practices. Ely and Thomas write:

> Inequality is bad for both business and society. Organizations limit their capacity for innovation and continuous improvement unless all employees are full participants in the enterprise: fully seen, heard, developed, engaged—and rewarded accordingly. Moreover, such treatment can unleash enormous reserves of leadership potential too long suppressed by systems that perpetuate inequality.[20]

Other thought leaders have called for organizations to move beyond diversity and inclusion initiatives toward advancing equity and eliminating systemic racism in the workplace as well as advancing efforts that promote racial healing and transformation.[19,23] Addressing bias and eliminating racist policies and procedures involve more than offering a diversity training program to all employees. Kalev and Dobbin suggest that an organization cannot affect bias simply with a series of antibias or awareness-level trainings.[24] Organizations today, especially public health agencies rooted in their missions to address health equity and promote optimal health for all, must undertake both internal work to undo systemic racism and external action to address health disparities and equity issues in their communities. Key to leveraging diversity and supporting inclusion on teams and within an organization overall are intentional, well-developed all-staff efforts to address racism and discrimination. In the communities that public health agencies serve, this includes adopting a racial healing and transformation approach to future work.[19]

Trust: The Secret Ingredient of Effective Teams

Studies of team efficacy find that trust is essential to effective teamwork. Along with different identities and complementary skills, high-performing teams require trust among their ranks. In his best-selling management fable *The Five Dysfunctions of a Team*, Patrick Lencioni describes the role trust plays in promoting team performance and, by extension, generating better results for an organization.[25] Andy Molinsky and Ernest Gundling write about the importance of trust to the performance of cross-cultural teams, calling trust the glue that holds an effective team together.[26] Stephen M. R. Covey describes the importance of trust in creating effective business relationships and allowing organizations to move at the "speed of trust" to accomplish goals more effectively and efficiently.[27] In an article on resilient teams and COVID-19, Stoverink and colleagues found that more resilient teams also had more trust among their members, in addition to several other characteristics, such as being able to improvise, sharing a mental model of teamwork, and believing they could effectively complete tasks together.[28]

Trusting relationships are built on vulnerability, and baring this vulnerability allows for team cohesion and shared understanding. Without trust, individual team members may feel unsafe taking risks or developing innovations, may shy away from conflict, and may lack commitment to shared goals or results.[25] In Lencioni's model, lack of commitment leads to avoidance of accountability and failure to reach shared goals because not all members may buy into the team's work or be committed to its success. Team members who exhibit vulnerability share their views and perspectives or suggest alternatives to complex problems one team member may be unable to solve alone, bringing their diverse experience, viewpoints, and expertise to the task.

Deliberation and debate are essential to high-performing teams and should take place in a "safe space" afforded by trust and free of bias or discrimination. In organizations lacking trust, even the most diverse team may have members who shut down or otherwise refuse to share their viewpoints because they are unsure of the group's commitment. Therefore, organizations looking to optimize team performance must identify systemic racism and other discrimination at work and commit to the work of racial healing, including changing organizational policies and procedures that may implicitly advantage one group over another. Without these efforts, trust cannot be fully developed or sustained, and diversity and inclusion efforts are unlikely to generate the impact they otherwise could have on organizational performance.

Summary

Business administration, management, and organizational development literature points to the value of diversity and inclusion, especially work by diverse and inclusive teams, to high-performing organizations. The business and moral cases for diversity and inclusion reveal internal and external benefits that diverse teams of public health practitioners can yield for their organizations and their jurisdictions—especially when leaders create and sustain trusting workplace cultures. As one of the nine critical strategic skills, diversity and inclusion, as well as support for racial healing and transformation efforts, should be part of every public health practitioner's toolkit.

References

1. Jonathan Vespa, Lauren Medina, and David M. Armstrong, "Demographic Turning Points for the United States: Population Projections for 2020 to 2060," U.S. Census Bureau, *Population Estimates and Projects, Current Population Reports*, 25–114, https://www.census.gov/content/dam/Census/library/publications/2020/demo/p25-1144.pdf.
2. Dennis W. Pullin, "Taking My Shot at Building Trust," *Modern Healthcare*, December 29, 2020, https://www.modernhealthcare.com/opinion-editorial/taking-my-shot-building-trust.
3. Nina Feldman, "Why the Head of the Black Doctors COVID-19 Consortium Decided to Get Vaccinated," WHYY, December 16, 2020, https://whyy.org/articles/why-the-head-of-the-black-doctors-covid-19-consortium-decided-to-get-vaccinated/.
4. "2021 PH WINS Dashboards," de Beaumont Foundation, https://www.phwins.org/national.
5. "Top Executive Characteristics (Profile of Local Health Departments)," National Association of County and City Health Officials (NACCHO), https://www.naccho.org/profile-report-dashboard/leadership.
6. National Consortium for Public Health Workforce Development, *Building Skills for a More Strategic Public Health Workforce: A Call to Action,*

de Beaumont Foundation, https://www.debeaumont.org/wp-content/uploads/2019/04/Building-Skills-for-a-More-Strategic-Public-Health-Workforce.pdf.

7. "Center for State and Local Government Excellence Identifies Six State and Local Workforce Trends to Watch in 2021," *PR Newswire*, December 31, 2020, https://www.prnewswire.com/news-releases/center-for-state-and-local-government-excellence-identifies-six-workforce-trends-to-watch-in-2021-301199666.html.

8. Center for State and Local Government Excellence (SLGE), "Stakeholders Meeting on Developing the Public Sector Workforce of the Future," https://slge.org/resources/stakeholders-report-developing-the-public-sector-workforce-of-the-future.

9. Chazeman S. Jackson and J. Nadine Gracia, "Addressing Health and Health-care Disparities: The Role of a Diverse Workforce and the Social Determinants of Health," *Public Health Reports* 129, suppl. 2 (2014): 57–61.

10. Jon R. Katzenbach and Douglas K. Smith, "The Discipline of Teams," *Harvard Business Review* March-April 1993, https://hbr.org/1993/03/the-discipline-of-teams-2.

11. Jon Katzenbach and Douglas Smith, *The Wisdom of Teams: Creating the High-Performance Organization* (Boston, MA: Harvard Business Review Press, 2015).

12. Scott E. Page, *The Diversity Bonus: How Great Teams Pay Off in the Knowledge Economy* (Princeton, NJ: Princeton University Press, 2017), https://www.jstor.org/stable/j.ctvc77fcqhttps://www.jstor.org/stable/j.ctvc77fcq.

13. Vivian Hunt, David Layton, and Sara Prince, "Why Diversity Matters," McKinsey & Company, 2015, https://www.mckinsey.com/~/media/McKinsey/Business%20Functions/Organization/Our%20Insights/Why%20diversity%20matters/Why%20diversity%20matters.pdf.

14. Katherine W. Phillips, "How Diversity Makes Us Smarter," *Scientific American*, October 2014, https://www.scientificamerican.com/article/how-diversity-makes-us-smarter.

15. David Rock and Heidi Grant, "Why Diverse Teams Are Smarter," *Harvard Business Review*, November 4, 2016 https://hbr.org/2016/11/why-diverse-teams-are-smarter.

16. Catherine C. Eckel and Phillip J. Grossman, "Managing Diversity by Creating Team Identity," *Journal of Economic Behavior & Organization* 58, no. 3 (2005): 271–392, https://www.sciencedirect.com/science/article/abs/pii/S0167268104002070.

17. Anna Johansson, "The One Philosophical Difference That Set Millennials Apart in Workplace Diversity," *Forbes*, November 13, 2017,

https://www.forbes.com/sites/annajohansson/2017/11/13/the-one-philos
ophical-difference-that-sets-millennials-apart-in-workplace-divers
ity/?sh=2f51a98970c7.

18. Fabian Homberg and Hong T. M. Bui, "Top Management Team
Diversity: A Systematic Review," *Group & Organizational Management* 38,
no. 4 (2013): 455–479, https://journals.sagepub.com/doi/10.1177/10596
01113493925.

19. *Truth, Racial Healing & Transformation Implementation Guidebook*, W.K.
Kellogg Foundation, December 2016, https://healourcommunities.org/
wp-content/uploads/2018/02/TRHTImplementationGuide.pdf.

20. Robin J. Ely and David A. Thomas, "Getting Serious About Diversity:
Enough Already with the Business Case," *Harvard Business Review*,
November/December 2020, 2020. https://hbr.org/2020/11/getting-seri
ous-about-diversity-enough-already-with-the-business-case.

21. David A. Thomas and Robin J. Ely, "Making Differences Matter: A New
Paradigm for Managing Diversity," *Harvard Business Review*, September/
October 1996, https://hbr.org/1996/09/making-differences-matter-a-
new-paradigm-for-managing-diversity.

22. Carmen Morris, "Anti-Racism: Why Your DEI Agenda Will Never Be a
Success without It," *Forbes*, December 15, 2020, https://www.forbes.
com/sites/carmenmorris/2020/12/15/anti-racism-why-your-dei-agenda-
will-never-be-a-success-without-it.

23. Ben Hecht, "Moving Beyond Diversity Toward Racial Equity," *Harvard
Business Review*, June 16, 2020, https://hbr.org/2020/06/moving-beyond-
diversity-toward-racial-equity.

24. Alexandra Kalev and Frank Dobbin, "Companies Need to Think Bigger
Than Diversity Training," *Harvard Business Review*, October 20, 2020,
https://hbr.org/2020/10/companies-need-to-think-bigger-than-divers
ity-training.

25. Patrick Lencioni, *The Five Dysfunctions of a Team: A Leadership Fable* (San
Francisco, CA: Jossey-Bass, 2002).

26. Andy Molinsky and Ernest Gundling, "How to Build Trust on Your
Cross-cultural Team," *Harvard Business Review*, June 28, 2016, https://
hbr.org/2016/06/how-to-build-trust-on-your-cross-cultural-team.

27. Stephen M. R. Covey, *Speed of Trust: The One Thing That Changes
Everything* (New York: The Free Press, 2006).

28. Adam C. Stoverink et al., "Bouncing Back Together: Toward a
Theoretical Model of Work Team Resilience," *Academy of Management
Review* 45, no. 2 (2020): 395–422, https://journals.aom.org/doi/
abs/10.5465/amr.2017.0005.

Growing Strategic Skills to Support Innovation in Governmental Public Health

JESSICA SOLOMON FISHER, REENA CHUDGAR, AND GRACE CASTILLO

THE BUSINESS SECTOR—WITH ITS EXPECTATIONS of remaining relevant and viable—relies on innovation. Governmental public health is not a business in the traditional sense; it does not aim to make a profit, to increase sales, or to attract more customers. In fact, pursuing the goals of public health—to serve all, to prevent disease, to achieve equity, and more—results in fewer customers. Yet, despite this seemingly divergent agenda, adopting a business innovation mindset can unleash public health's ability to be agile and responsive to changing community needs, to use real-time information and data, and to engage with existing or new partners to amplify reach.

The need for innovation in governmental public health practice is clear, yet innovation is not a mindset that historically has been taught in schools of public health nor particularly fostered in practice. In thinking about the skills needed to work effectively in public health today, cultivating a culture of innovation is of utmost importance.

Jessica Solomon Fisher, Reena Chudgar, and Grace Castillo, *Growing Strategic Skills to Support Innovation in Governmental Public Health* In: *Building Strategic Skills for Better Health: A Primer for Public Health Professionals.* Edited by: Michael R. Fraser and Brian C. Castrucci, Oxford University Press. © de Beaumont Foundation 2024. DOI: 10.1093/oso/9780197744604.003.0015

Emerging and recurring health threats mandate both rapid response and the infrastructure necessary to support this response, as well as the need to plan strategically and innovatively to get ahead of the threats. We need new ways of addressing immediate and longer-term public health priorities. In short, we ought to be asking ourselves: What is the public health equivalent of the iPhone? How can we solve the complex, interrelated problems driving health inequities? iPhones aren't the answer, but if public health adopts an innovation mindset and grows agencies that foster creativity, we open the door to asking the right questions and finding more effective answers. By collaborating with communities, we can co-produce solutions with a stronger impact. This is the power of innovation.

Public health has increasingly responded to the dynamic world around it, addressing issues that previously were considered outside of traditional practice. It has embraced concepts such as Public Health 3.0, a model that designates public health leaders as "health strategists" who partner with multiple sectors and leverage data to address social and economic conditions that affect health.[1] The competencies and skills needed to work in, and to lead, health departments have changed.[2] As a result, we need to look to how our leaders and teams are developing a culture of innovation, creating new programs, and embracing an innovation mindset and skill set. Governmental public health must increase its focus on innovation and infuse it into workplace culture. We have done it before: vaccines, the use of mobile technology for health communication and tracking, the development and use of Incident Command Structure to manage emergency and disaster response, and the adoption of a quality mindset in public health are just a handful of public health's innovation success stories.

What Is Innovation in Public Health?

Renowned biochemist Albert Szent-Gyorgyi said, "Innovation is seeing what everybody has seen and thinking what nobody has thought."[3] In its simplest terms, innovation isn't doing things better, it's doing better things. Innovation can be more than a buzzword. Innovation processes and mindsets can be powerful tools in transforming public health practice to address complex problems and to grow its role in working with partners and the community to improve population health and equity. For business and other sectors, innovation is about doing something new to boost the bottom line, to improve results, to improve quality, or to pivot to meet changing customer needs. For public health, innovation is about more, given the mission to prevent illness, to improve health and well-being, and to achieve equity. To that end, public health innovation[4] can be defined as the creation and implementation of a novel process, policy, product, program, or system leading to improvements that impact health and equity. Tenets of public health innovation include:

- It is an ongoing, systematic process that can generate incremental or radical change.
- It requires both collaboration with diverse team members and partners and co-production with people with lived experience who will be affected by the results of the innovation.
- It is an open process that lends itself to adaptation or replication.

Despite the common misperception that innovation means throwing lots of ideas against the wall and seeing what sticks, a systematic process underpins the approach. This process helps create meaningful solutions in conjunction with the communities that health departments serve. In public health, an example of innovation could be a new program or tool to address equity. Or it could take the form of internal focus on creating a new business practice within a health department. While innovation is not the answer to every public health problem, the process helps us ask the right questions and find the right solutions, keeping communities at the center throughout. Innovation is not just an additional task added to day-to-day work; it requires a shift in the way we approach our work. Public health must reimagine traditional tactical skills and develop a collation of more strategic skills.

The World Economic Forum's *The Future of Jobs Report 2018* cited analytical thinking and innovation, active learning and learning strategies, and creativity, originality, and initiative as the skills in greatest demand and need for 2022.[5] The American Management

Association's *Critical Skills Survey* found that critical thinking and problem-solving, effective communication, collaboration and team-building, and creativity and innovation were becoming increasingly important.[6] Common to these lists and the strategic skills described in this book are themes that underlie building or maintaining an organizational culture that supports innovation. In addition to the variety of skills needed in public health practice, the following concepts are fundamental to providing space for leaders and staff to move from doing things "the way they have always been done" to embracing innovation as a tool to help improve communities:

- Empathy is at the heart of innovation. Innovation processes are human-centered, and innovation seeks to understand how the user experiences a problem and where there are pain points. Empathy is about taking time to develop a deep understanding of what is important to people, being curious, and understanding nuances of a problem people are facing. Through empathy, we can create a connection with people, with communities, and with the system, all of which can motivate creativity and lead to innovation. Empathy in innovation is about "walking in another's shoes" and can manifest itself in public health through authentic community engagement. Through valuing the community's experience and perspective in decision-making, whether on individual solutions to problems or in processes like community health improvement planning, empathy is a bedrock of innovation.
- Risk-taking is essential to innovation. As stewards of public funds within a regulatory structure, government staff hesitate to take risks. Yet the nature of innovation is about working in uncertainty, albeit in a controlled, systemized environment. Public health practice tells us to use the evidence base—which we should do when proven, effective interventions are available. When no such solution exists, we can use innovation to help create an evidence base rather than spend valuable resources planning for what might be the wrong question or solution. A culture of innovation supports staff in taking risks without fear of penalty. Workplace leaders must create this

culture of challenging the status quo, championing those who take risks, and embracing both failures and successes. In public health, this could be the small-scale implementation of a new educational campaign that has not been tested but holds promise because it was developed through an innovation process that engaged the end user. It could be using a new technology platform to elicit community engagement in planning processes or testing expanded roadway walking lanes during the COVID-19 pandemic.

- Failure. With all endeavors, failure is a possibility. Failure often provides rich learnings that benefit the innovation process, but it still is seen as undesirable and may be met with negative consequences. Design and innovation expert David Kelley, founder of IDEO, says, "Fail faster to succeed sooner."[7] The design thinking process allows for early failure in small ways that don't waste time or money, making it an effective tool for making failure safe. One example is prototyping, a key and generative step in the design thinking process that ameliorates risk by testing, evaluating, and learning to inform future iterations of the innovation. The prototyping step minimizes lost time and money spent on implementing the wrong solutions. And the concept of failing forward is about learning from failures to create the best success possible. In innovation processes, we succeed even when the solution we implement doesn't work because we learn and improve based on failure.[8] Creating a culture where failure, and failing forward, are encouraged is essential to innovation. Failing gives us room to learn. The idea of having personal cell phones serve more or less as computers resulted in the iPhone and Android phones, products on which many of us rely heavily. But before they launched, there were the Simon Personal Communicator, BlackBerry, and Palm Pilot, none of which succeeded but all of which were innovations that sparked a movement toward the smartphone revolution.
- Creativity. Although innovation and creativity overlap, true innovation is applied, practical, and hands-on, with a focus

on implementation. Creativity, which informs innovation, is about the conception of the ideas themselves. As an input to innovation, creativity requires creating a space for staff and leaders to be imaginative in their everyday work—it requires time and space to think beyond the way things have always been done. Creativity flourishes when we consistently question what could be, are alert to possibility in unsolved problems, and continuously try to shift perspective to open new ways of thinking. Using a public health approach to prevent violence,[9] asking a fast-food manager about how to manage drive-through COVID vaccination sites,[10] and developing an online community health improvement planning process are all examples of how creativity is an integral element of innovation.

- Co-production is a form of community engagement where the end user, or person with lived experience, is an active participant and driver of the innovation process. In its truest form, this means that a health department engages end users to ideate, test, implement, and design. Co-production is at the heart of community health improvement planning. It allows us to understand the issues at hand more deeply and ultimately to create solutions with the community. If we don't dig deep enough—asking communities how they have adapted to their circumstances and what creative workarounds they have invented—we cannot understand how a given community experiences a problem. We also cannot help to solve that problem in a meaningful way. Whether for community health improvement planning or the development of other programming that is in direct response to community needs, health departments are accustomed to working with communities. Co-production deepens community engagement, calling on the expertise of community members to develop solutions.

- Change management. If innovation is about empathy, perhaps it goes without saying that innovation and change management go hand in hand. Change management is a tool best employed to help organizations undergoing a change in approach or culture, such as adopting an innovation mindset and fostering a movement toward that culture. Addressing the human side of change to understand how this shift impacts employees helps staff lend their support to, and participate in, changes to the status quo. (For additional information on change management, see chapters 4 and 5.)

Innovation itself is not a skill but a mindset and a way of thinking. Innovation exists in the bigger context of the environment that surrounds it, and it is important in systems thinking; systems thinking is also important to innovation. Innovation should take into account all of the aspects and connectivity of a system—people, processes, structures, and more. Systems thinking and innovation also both strive to get to the root of a problem, to understand the current state and connectivity of things, to identify patterns, and to discern why things are the way they are. While innovation comes naturally to some, for others it's an area they can develop when given an environment primed to support innovative processes. For instance, a systems thinker grasps patterns and relationships to understand systems contributing to public health problems and identifies high-impact interventions. This ability to see beyond a single data point to how people, programs, and problems feed back into each other is essential to innovation. It supports looking at the whole and the parts, comprehensively, to create transformative, radical, or disruptive solutions.

For innovation to take root, an organization must place as much value on these skills as it does on technical public health skills. Health department leaders must facilitate innovation cultures, allowing the mindset to grow. However, leaders must also consider how to develop these skills in the workforce. What incremental changes can be infused to support innovation in the existing workforce? What more radical changes can we make to encourage the emerging workforce to innovate? As innovation in the field flourishes, schools of public health and other related sectors should teach these strategic skills as standard practice, to build the foundation for innovation.

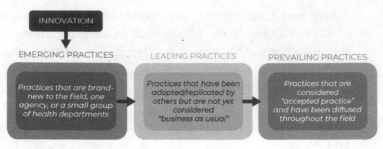

Figure 14.1. Innovation.

Below, we discuss where the public health is currently when it comes to strategic skills (figure 14.1).

Data from the Public Health Workforce Interests and Needs Survey

Public health must increase its support of creativity and innovation. Data from the 2021 Public Health Workforce Interests and Needs Survey (PH WINS), the only nationally representative survey of the governmental public health workforce, found that only 46% of health department workers felt their workplace rewarded creativity and innovation. In some health departments, that number was as low as 22%.[11] Although this may not seem like a problem at first glance, supporting innovation plays a critical role in building more effective organizations with experienced staff. As the 2021 PH WINS data showed, 27% of public health practitioners were considering leaving their job in the upcoming year, with 22% of the total workforce planning departures for reasons other than retirement.[11]

Supporting innovation can address this impending problem. Actively valuing innovation and creativity impacts the top reasons practitioners cite when leaving the field—workplace environment, job satisfaction, inadequate pay, and lack of support. Practitioners who felt that their organization supported innovation showed greater job and workplace satisfaction than those who did not feel that way. These practitioners were also twice as likely to be satisfied with their pay—a major finding in a field where inadequate pay has long been a contentious issue.

Clearly, fostering innovation is one of the best investments the field can make. But how can public health organizations begin to make these overdue changes? A host of structural issues, discussed in the case examples below, can hamper innovation. However, organizations still have substantial control over their workplace environment. One way to encourage innovation is simply to expect it and to communicate this expectation to practitioners. Currently, only 29% of workers strongly agree that they're expected to be creative or to think of new ways to do things at work.[12] Explicitly adding innovation as a part of performance is a powerful way to shift this perception and to encourage innovation. Workplaces may also benefit from training in change management to address the challenges that come with any effort to change organizational culture. Recognizing innovation's benefits, the field must build organizations and workplace environments that better support this approach. Practitioners, public health, and our communities will all benefit.

Examples of Innovation in Public Health

Structural and historical barriers exist that prevent public health from innovating. First, public health extends into nearly every sector, including business and social services. Governmental public health systems extend across local, state, national, and federal levels. These layers and systems are interconnected, impact one another, and influence the way public health work is accomplished, such as disease- or intervention-specific funding streams. This structure makes uniform fixes unworkable and mandates thinking beyond one data point and taking a systems approach to solving problems. Second, public health values evidence-based solutions and has historically relied on evidence-based practices in addressing a problem. Innovations take a while to make it into the evidence base. While innovation's benefits are indisputable, it necessarily takes a forward-looking approach that may feel risky. Finally, all innovation carries a substantial risk of failure. This uncertainty can be uncomfortable, especially when the status quo seems predictable and workable and public funds are at stake.

Even in the face of these challenges, some public health agencies are prioritizing innovation. The discussion that follows outlines five examples.

Case Study: Garrett County Health Department, Maryland

Tom Freston, cofounder of MTV, said, "Innovation is taking two things that exist and putting them together in a new way." Think of how putting wheels on a suitcase changed the way we travel. Now think about how an online, open-source tool could change the way we engage in community health improvement planning. That is exactly what happened in Garrett County, Maryland. The Garrett County Health Department, seeking to comprehensively reflect the complexity of local health issues and to increase participation in the assessment planning process such that priorities better reflect all residents, developed the Universal Community Planning Tool (UCPT). Recognizing that traditional outreach approaches like public meetings were not capturing sufficient resident input, particularly from vulnerable populations, the health department moved its process online. The UCPT allows data collection, measure development and tracking, community forums for residents to discuss concerns and develop priorities, and more. The approach and open-source nature of the tool are so compelling that health departments across the country have adopted it and have created their own online outreach resources to improve community engagement.[13]

Case Study: Chicago, Illinois

Thomas Edison said, "The value of an idea lies in the using of it." When the University of Illinois at Chicago and the Chicago Department of Public Health realized that there was no mechanism to understand whether public funds were appropriately matched to community health needs, they worked to utilize publicly available data to analyze the distribution of funds for health and health-related human services within the City of Chicago. The team developed a process and open-source platform that health departments and other government agencies can use to assess whether public funds are spatially matched to community health needs.[14]

Case Study: DuPage County Health Department, Illinois

Economist Theodore Levitt said, "Creativity is thinking up new things. Innovation is doing new things." The Post-Crisis Response Team (PCRT) in DuPage County, Illinois, is a cross-sector partnership designed to address the mental health needs of individuals involved in the criminal justice system by providing linkages to behavioral health treatment and other social service resources. It is a collaboration between the DuPage County Health Department and DuPage County Sheriff's Office. The PCRT follows up on any 911 call with a mental health component and refers individuals to mental and social services as needed. The project utilizes data refinement to streamline the crime-reporting codes used to identify 911 calls with a mental health component.[15]

Case Study: Tacoma-Pierce County Health Department, Washington

Steven Johnson, science author and media theorist, said, "If you look at history, innovation doesn't come just from giving people incentives; it comes from creating environments where their ideas can connect." In Pierce County, Washington, the health department looked for a way to engage residents more meaningfully in public health and local government decision-making. After considering more traditional approaches, the agency realized it needed to shift control of the decision-making process away from government and toward empowering the community, to promote social cohesion and self-efficacy among residents, and to support equitable distribution of resources through participatory budgeting. After a pilot with the parks department, the agency worked with three schools in underserved communities within the county, engaging students and parents in making decisions about allocating funds to improve aspects of the schools. This project highlights an important part of successful innovation: collaboration between diverse entities. By opening up the budgeting process to new stakeholders—stakeholders with a relevant, knowledgeable perspective—budgeting became more responsive, targeted, and transparent.[16]

Case Study: Ohio Department of Health

Albert Einstein said that we can't solve our problems by using the same kind of thinking we used when we created them. Establishing flexible and sustainable cross-sector funding models to address Ohio's emerging and most pressing health issues is a strategic priority for the Ohio Department of Health. To that end, two new funding mechanisms were established as part of the state's 2020–2021 biennial budget.

The first is a commitment of $6 million to create a public health fund (PHF) that aligns with the governor's priorities and the State Health Improvement Plan. To ensure flexibility, the fund exists outside of state government, with a governance structure that includes state agency representatives and governor appointees as board members. The PHF issues grants and conducts projects that offer innovative, public–private approaches to the state's most pressing needs; that incubate programs at the local level that can be scalable; and that foster evidence-informed approaches in local programming. The awards are issued from interest earned on the initial investment, ensuring the fund's continuity.

The second mechanism is a separate new line of funding that will be available to state agencies, local health departments, and their community partners. The funds will be used to develop, implement, and evaluate innovative approaches to addressing State Health Improvement Plan priorities, with emphasis on the underlying community conditions that impact overall health and well-being.

Conclusion

Increasingly, innovation is an essential component of successful public health practice and improving health and equity. Although today's workplace, educational, and training systems need innovation, the landscape is rapidly changing. As we move toward systems approaches to solving public health issues, we must ensure that our workforce has the appropriate and relevant skills to undertake challenges and to develop innovative solutions. This starts with openness to change and willingness to support creativity and innovation in the workplace—something the workforce longs for. As the field looks to grow strategic skills and to cultivate leaders who support innovation, bright spots like the case studies above can serve as inspiration. These examples help build the repository of tools and resources needed to move emerging innovations into prevailing practices in public health. Ultimately, innovation will unlock our power to transform communities and to promote health for all.

References

1. "Public Health 3.0: A Call to Action to Create a 21st Century Public Health Infrastructure," U.S. Department of Health and Human Services, Office of the Assistant Secretary for Health, 2016, https://www.health ypeople.gov/sites/default/files/Public-Health-3.0-White-Paper.pdf.
2. Craig Tower et al., "Building Collective Efficacy to Support Public Health Workforce Development," *Journal of Public Health Management and Practice* 27, no. 1 (2021): 55–61, https://pubmed.ncbi.nlm.nih.gov/30969275/.
3. David Fairhurst, "Discovery Is Seeing What Everyone Else Has Seen—But Thinking What No One Else Has Thought," *HR Magazine*, February 17, 2012, https://www.hrmagazine.co.uk/content/features/discovery-is-seeing-what-everyone-else-has-seen-but-thinking-what-no-one-else-has-thought/.
4. "About Innovations—What Is Public Health Innovation?," The Public Health National Center for Innovation, https://phnci.org/innovations/about-innovations.
5. *The Future of Jobs Report 2018* (Geneva, Switzerland: World Economic Forum, 2018), http://www3.weforum.org/docs/WEF_Future_of_Jobs_2 018.pdf.
6. American Management Association staff, "AMA Critical Skills Survey: Workers Need Higher Level Skills to Succeed in the 21st Century," January 24, 2019, https://www.amanet.org/articles/ama-critical-skills-survey-workers-need-higher-level-skills-to-succeed-in-the-21st-century/.
7. "Why You Should Talk Less and Do More," IDEO Design Thinking, October 30, 2013, https://designthinking.ideo.com/blog/why-you-sho uld-talk-less-and-do-more.
8. John C. Maxwell, *Falling Forward: Turning Mistakes into Stepping Stones for Success* (New York: HarperCollins, 2007).

9. "Saving Lives, Transforming Communities," Cure Violence Global, https://cvg.org/.

10. Alaa Elassar, "A Chick-Fil-A Manager Saved a Drive-thru COVID-19 Vaccination Clinic after Traffic Backed up," *CNN Online*, January 31, 2021, https://www.cnn.com/2021/01/31/us/chick-fil-a-drive-thru-covid-vaccine-trnd/index.html.

11. de Beaumont Foundation and Association of State and Territorial Health Officials, "PH WINS 2021: Dashboards," August 3, 2021, https://www.phwins.org/national.

12. Ben Wigert and Jennifer Robison, "Fostering Creativity at Work: Do Your Managers Push or Crush Innovation?" *Gallup*, December 19, 2018, https://www.gallup.com/workplace/245498/fostering-creativity-work-managers-push-crush-innovation.aspx.

13. *Universal Community Planning Tool (UCPT) Project—Case Study Report*, The Public Health National Center for Innovations and NORC at The University of Chicago, February 2019, https://phnci.org/uploads/resource-files/PHNCI-Case-Study-Garrett-County.pdf.

14. *Next Generation Health and Human Services Infrastructure: A Process & Platform—A Case Study Report*, Public Health National Center for Innovations and The University of Chicago, April 2019, https://phnci.org/uploads/resource-files/PHNCI-Case-Study-University-of-Chicago.pdf.

15. *Post-Crisis Response Team (PCRT) Project—A Case Study Report*, Public Health National Center for Innovations and The University of Chicago, January 2019, https://phnci.org/uploads/resource-files/PHNCI-Case-Study-DuPage-County.pdf.

16. *Adopting Anticipatory Budgeting in Pierce County, Washington—A Case Study Report*, Public Health National Center for Innovations and The University of Chicago, April 2019, https://phnci.org/uploads/resource-files/PHNCI-Case-Study-Tacoma-Pierce-County.pdf.

15

STRATEGIC SKILLS IN FOCUS:
- ▶ *Policy Engagement*
- ▶ *Community Engagement*
- ▶ *Cross-Sectoral Partnerships*

Overview: Moving from Programs to Policies

The Public Health Professional as Advocate

EDWARD L. HUNTER AND GRACE CASTILLO

Introduction

The field of public health has always adapted to meet new challenges and to incorporate new approaches and technologies. Working at the community level to improve the fundamental conditions in which people live has long been an essential part of public health, exemplified by successes such as lead paint removal, tobacco control, and food and motor vehicle safety measures. More recently, public health advocates have amplified the importance of broader, more systemic approaches—including policy change—as they seek greater influence over social and economic circumstances that affect health, as well as sustainable interventions in the face of resource constraints. Prioritizing policy represents a paradigm shift within the field, and advocates have promoted making health an explicit consideration in a range of public policies to improve health outcomes and overall well-being.

Edward L. Hunter and Grace Castillo, *Overview: Moving from Programs to Policies* In: *Building Strategic Skills for Better Health: A Primer for Public Health Professionals*. Edited by: Michael R. Fraser and Brian C. Castrucci, Oxford University Press. © de Beaumont Foundation 2024. DOI: 10.1093/oso/9780197744604.003.0016

The United States' experience addressing the COVID-19 pandemic brought to the fore the importance of, and need for, effective use of policy levers to build more equitable and resilient communities, to control infectious diseases, to mitigate the impacts of health emergencies, and to protect public health science. The COVID-19 crisis made it clear that stepping back from policy engagement is not an option for those working to improve the public's health.

This chapter provides an overview of how advocates and practitioners can elevate policy as a public health tool—by shifting to a new paradigm in which policy skills and approaches make the field more strategic, impactful, and sustainable.

Policy in the Public Health Context

Public health policy involves using laws, regulations, and other instruments of government to achieve public health goals (box 15.1). Among other things, policy uses the inherent powers of government to impact the conditions in which people live, to encourage healthy practices by individuals and businesses, and to prohibit or discourage unhealthy products, practices, or behaviors.

BOX 15.1. DEFINITION OF POLICY

Policy is a term that is applied in multiple ways. Institutions can set policies to govern their own practices (e.g., how hospitals control infections, manage protection, or share patient data). Employers and health plans can establish policies that affect the working conditions and benefits of their employees and covered populations. Health systems (including those managed by governments) can implement policies that affect all of their member institutions, with wider impact. At the broadest level, laws, regulations, entitlements, and other measures adopted by governments— public policies—can have broad, sustainable impact and set a context for the actions of others in the community.

Source: Edward L. Hunter and Don Bradley, Overview—Policy: Achieving Sustained Impact, in *The Practical Playbook II: Building Multisector Partnerships That Work*, 2nd ed., eds. J. Lloyd Michener, Brian C. Castrucci, Don W. Bradley, Edward L. Hunter, Craig W. Thomas, Catherine Patterson, and Elizabeth Corcoran (New York: Oxford University Press), 385.

Public health services and programs often are supported by public funds and require consistent political support to sustain annual appropriations. Policies are designed to be durable—they are more likely to be in place for long periods without the need for renewed action. Political capital is necessary to enact major policies, and governments require funding to support implementation and enforcement of most policies, but policy interventions are unlikely to entail significant, long-term funding support. Programs and services usually target individuals, whereas policies target communities or populations. Policy interventions, therefore, are often preferred for their durability and efficiency.

As a tool, policy is not political or partisan, although support for a particular government intervention may reflect divisions between political ideologies. The use of policy as a public health intervention does require engagement in the political process, however. Laws are enacted by elected officials, and politically appointed administrators make the most significant regulatory decisions. Many public health practitioners shy away from seeking policy solutions because of an aversion to politics; however, much work in public health policy remains distant from the political fray. As the following sections of this chapter (and succeeding chapters) discuss, policy involves nonpartisan analysis, education, advocacy, and political engagement. Public health officials should not avoid policy simply because it is related to politics; rather, they should find the appropriate role and learn how to engage.[1] There are clear functions in public health advocacy that do not violate rules against lobbying, even by public officials or tax-exempt agencies.

This chapter examines public policy rather than policies enacted by private entities. Public health advocates can engage with governments at all levels, each of which has unique abilities to enact measures with broad impact on individual behavior and commercial activity. These include regulations and mandates (e.g., regulating tobacco or alcohol sales), taxes that raise revenue for programs but also incentivize or discourage behaviors by individuals and businesses, and spending measures for programs or more enduring infrastructure. All branches of government play a part: legislatures enact laws, executives implement and enforce them (often through legislatively empowered regulation), and courts interpret laws and regulations in the context of constitutional rights.

Shifting Public Health Goals Need Policy Solutions

Traditionally, public health as a field emphasized delivery of effective, evidence-based programs and services to individuals and communities. This required focus on appropriations advocacy to support a robust public health infrastructure and efforts to direct resources to the highest-value programs. A principal goal was to inform actions by healthcare professionals and institutions and to develop a workforce of skilled public health scientists to effectively manage public health programs.

The growing aspiration among advocates to influence events beyond public health's traditional domain requires a paradigm shift to greater reliance on policy as a public health tool. This more strategic approach to policy recognizes that public policies across a broad spectrum—both inside and outside the health field—are essential for improving health and well-being. This is a fundamental feature of the Health in All Policies movement,[1] which advocates for considering health impact across the full range of public policies.

Despite increased ambition and recognition of the importance of policy engagement, few governmental public health agencies have invested in developing policy capacity.[2] Many practitioners report being unaware of policy approaches like Health in All Policies, as well as a lack of skill and experience in developing policy.[3] To be more strategic, agencies and advocates must elevate the priority and resources given to policy in the public health workforce and emphasize that policy is a core responsibility of public health professionals. To improve the impact of policy engagement, these professionals also must work with other sectors in new ways to create innovative solutions to seemingly non-health-related policies that influence health (e.g., housing regulations and zoning decisions). This process will call on public health practitioners to gain the trust of cross-sectoral partners by engaging with them as peers and by carefully listening to their needs and priorities to create mutually beneficial and powerful policies. This new imperative seeks to:

- Understand broad social and economic influences on health and identify opportunities to use policy levers to address them
- Adapt public health evidence to real-world decisions in other sectors
- Bring public health concepts and evidence to bear on public policy decisions beyond the domain of public health and even beyond the health sector
- Identify a range of policy levers that may contribute to improving health and well-being
- Identify the motivations and influencers of decisions in other sectors, and the kinds of evidence that relate to their decisions
- Protect public health science from political interference and ensure that evidence generated by public health agencies is readily available to the public and decision makers

As public health's role in shaping policy grows, so does the mandate to clearly articulate the need for practitioners' involvement in this sphere. Applying a public health lens to housing regulations or zoning decisions may not be intuitive for people with experience in those sectors. Those professionals—many of whom have great expertise within their field—may view public health practitioners as seeking to usurp their role or feel disrespected by the notion that a new model is important. For these reasons, public health practitioners must understand the priorities of people in other sectors and gain their trust.

Targets for Public Health Policy Interventions

Effectiveness in policy requires public health officials and advocates to focus on new audiences. For the most part, public health traditionally has targeted evidence and advocacy to a primary audience that includes other public health officials, health professionals, sophisticated users of evidence, and partners.

The target audience for policy advocacy is different. Usually, it comprises elected officials and those who influence them, who are likely to be less familiar with science, public health concepts, or evidence as traditionally applied to public health programs. Other targets include leaders of influential community institutions who have connections and influence with policymakers. These targets are unlikely to share a common vocabulary, or even to recognize common goals, with public health advocates.

Influencing decision makers is a vital part of unleashing advocacy's potential. Although public health professionals value evidence, other concerns—like ideology, compelling stories, economic impact, and anecdotal evidence—sway legislative choices. Even though public health is an evidence-driven field, advocates should understand that evidence of health impact (or even the effectiveness of interventions) has its limits within the legislative realm.

Public health leaders also need to target officials and experts in other fields and disciplines to appeal to non-health decision makers and to form partnerships and coalitions that extend their reach. Regardless of how strong the evidence is, a proposed policy must garner support from multiple coalitions to be enacted. This requires understanding the "language" of other sectors and how public health concepts can be effectively translated and made relevant in new contexts. For instance, many gains in tobacco-control policy came through agencies that regulated commerce (instead of health per se) and required messaging in the business community that allayed concerns about lost revenue. Recent attempts to raise the smoking age to 21 took a different and more direct tack: "Passing T21 may seem like lost revenue, but a healthier workforce means lower healthcare costs and ultimate savings for the business sector."[3]

Policy Skills

As the goal of public health shifts toward wider policy engagement, the public health workforce needs to adapt. Public health professionals are a diverse group representing multiple disciplines and perspectives. There is no single profession that defines public health—the field draws on practitioners trained in medicine, epidemiology, statistics, biology, community health, and many other disciplines. The 2021 Public Health Workforce Interests and Needs Survey (PH WINS) demonstrates that less than 15% of the governmental public health workforce has academic training in public health.[4] Building policy capacity requires embracing policy as an essential skill—elevating the importance of policy within public health professions, hiring policy professionals in public health spaces, building policy training into academic and in-service training curricula, and cultivating greater policy awareness among public health leaders.

Effectiveness in the policy sphere requires moving away from a sole reliance on medical science and program management toward skills related to influencing and motivating the action of decision makers outside the health field. These skills include:

- Understanding non-health sectors that are the targets of public health policy advocacy
- Researching laws and regulations, including "legal and policy surveillance,"[5] and interacting with lawyers and legislative staff to translate public health goals into appropriate legal and administrative vehicles
- Conducting policy analysis, which CDC describes as the process of identifying potential options to address a problem and then comparing those options to choose the most effective, efficient, and feasible[6]
- Navigating basic concepts of federalism to identify opportunities at different levels of government, then identifying opportunities for replication in other jurisdictions
- Understanding legislative procedure and the dynamics of legislative bodies
- Understanding the political context in which public health works, including political, ideological, and other nonscientific influences on decision-making
- Developing partnerships and coalitions
- Undertaking advocacy, persuasion, communication, negotiation, and compromise
- Guiding implementation of adopted policies by helping translate provisions of law and regulation into public health practice
- Designing, executing, and evaluating policy interventions

Evidence Needed for Public Health Policy

Evidence is just as critical to the pursuit of policy as it is for other public health interventions. Policy advocacy builds on traditional public health evidence (e.g., understanding patterns of disease and health risks, assessment of effectiveness and return on investment) but relies on an expanded range of relevant evidence. Therefore, the field must expand the types of evidence it collects and prioritizes. While measurable health outcomes often are what public health practitioners default to, other types of evidence can make a more compelling case for action. Liquor store density provides a window into different types of valuable evidence: alcohol availability impacts health outcomes.[7] Rather than this health argument for limiting density, however, city officials might be more persuaded by evidence about the effect of reducing density on the financial impact of crime, leading them to consider changing zoning laws.[8] The result in each case—fewer liquor stores—is the same; the persuasive evidence is different. Are businesses uninterested in tobacco restrictions but concerned about employee healthcare costs? Are city planners focused on commute times? Depending on the stakeholders, public health should prioritize collecting and sharing certain types of evidence, including economic impact and effect on equity.

To design effective policies and inform strategies for adoption, public health professionals need to expand the information they gather to include:

- The relationship between specific policy choices and health outcomes, identifying priority targets for policy advocacy and making the case that policy change will have an impact
- Distribution of costs and returns to specific players (and how these are related to constituents of elected officials) in coalitions of support or opposition and for designing tax or other financing mechanisms
- Projected economic impact, including tax revenue, jobs, economic mobility, and income security of affected communities, as these are important considerations in adopting and implementing a proposed policy

- Estimated time horizon for results in relation to elected officials' terms of office or tenure of other decision makers

Conclusion

A strategic policy approach for public health can reach beyond measures under the direct control of public health agencies or elsewhere in the health sector. Policy gets at the non-healthcare influencers of health, like housing, food access, and stable employment, all increasingly important targets of public health attention. Regulations and laws reach millions, can promote equity, and may bring lasting change to people's lives. Public health cannot and should not be the sole influence on policy, but effective, relevant advocacy and cross-sector communication are essential to advancing public health goals. This expands public health's reach and makes for better, more tailored policies.

Pursuing policy change is not without challenges. Policy skills are outside the training or experience of many practitioners, and restrictions on "lobbying" can be hard to interpret or apply in real-world situations. The use of governmental powers can invite opposition from those whose economic or political interests are affected (such as businesses subject to mandates, those whose tax burden is changed, or those who oppose extending government further into American life). Each of these challenges should be approached with a carefully designed strategy, skilled communications, and evidence of effectiveness. By making policy a strategic priority, public health practitioners and advocates can have real influence outside the health sector and help shape the broad social and economic conditions that are fundamental to improving the public's health.

References

1. Edward L. Hunter, "Politics and Public Health—Engaging the Third Rail," *Journal of Public Health Management and Practice* 22, no. 5 (2016): 436–441, https://www.ncbi.nlm.nih.gov/pmc/articles/PMC4974059/.
2. "Key Findings of PH WINS 2017," de Beaumont Foundation, https://deb eaumont.org/signup-phwins/findings/.
3. American Public Health Association, Public Health Institute, and California Department of Public Health, "Health in All Policies: A Guide

for State and Local Governments," 2013, https://www.apha.org/topics-and-issues/health-in-all-policies.

4. Institute of Medicine (US), Committee on Assuring the Health of the Public in the 21st Century, "Employers and Business," in *The Future of the Public's Health in the 21st Century* (Washington, DC: National Academies Press, 2002), https://www.ncbi.nlm.nih.gov/books/NBK221235/.
5. "PH WINS 2021: Explore the Data," de Beaumont Foundation, https://phwins.org/national.
6. Geresom Ilukor, "Challenges in the Implementation and Enforcement of Environmental Health and Public Health Law by Environmental Health Workers in Uganda: A Systematic Review," *International Journal of Health Sciences and Research* 9, no. 4 (2019): 242.
7. "Policy Analysis," Office of the Associate Director for Policy and Strategy, Centers for Disease Control and Prevention, revised March 2, 2021, https://www.cdc.gov/policy/polaris/policyprocess/policyanalysis/index.html.
8. Yi Lu, Pamela Trangenstein, and David H. Jernigan, "Policy-maker Relevant Metrics to Break the Link Between Alcohol Outlets and Violence" (presentation, American Public Health Association 2020 Virtual Annual Meeting and Expo, October 24–28, 2020).

16

Policy Development and Engagement

Turning Evidence into Action

KATRINA FORREST AND SHELLEY HEARNE

PUBLIC HEALTH PRACTITIONERS WORK ON the front lines of local, state, and federal government to protect and improve the health of individuals and communities. From epidemiologists to emergency responders, public health nurses to program managers, practitioners often face challenges with significant policy implications. The COVID-19 pandemic exposed the fragility of our public health infrastructure and exacerbated long-standing health inequities. As the United States contends with the coronavirus and its acute and chronic impacts on health and well-being, more than ever public health professionals should be engaged in policy efforts to improve the nation's emergency response and long-term resiliency.

Policy is one of our most powerful tools for improving people's lives. The public health field can enhance its impact and effectiveness by knowing how to develop and advocate for evidence-based policy solutions. While public health excels in assessment, analysis,

Katrina Forrest and Shelley Hearne, *Policy Development and Engagement* In: *Building Strategic Skills for Better Health: A Primer for Public Health Professionals.* Edited by: Michael R. Fraser and Brian C. Castrucci, Oxford University Press. © de Beaumont Foundation 2024. DOI: 10.1093/oso/9780197744604.003.0017 and analytical skills, we need to ensure that the facts, data, and research generated by the field are used to inform policymaking decisions. Moving evidence into action, however, can be a daunting task. For instance, over the past decade, state vaccination laws have been severely weakened despite evidence that reducing community immunity would put many vulnerable populations at risk. Political, emotional, and irrational fears drove decision-making. How do we adequately inform and appropriately engage with decision makers so that our evidence-based, expertise-based, or experience-based policy solutions become realities?

This chapter aims to equip public health professionals and all who seek to advocate for evidence-based policy solutions with tangible tools, skills, and insights necessary for achieving a policy objective.

Policy Development

In the seminal series *The Future of the Public's Health in the 21st Century*, the Academy of Medicine identified three core functions of public health practice: assessment of health status and health needs, assurance that necessary services are provided, and policy development.[1] Generally speaking, policy development is the process of developing policy through extensive research, analysis, consultation with stakeholders, and synthesis of the collected information to form actionable recommendations. Policies can be laws, regulations, procedures, administrative actions (including budget allocations), incentives, or voluntary practices of governments and other institutions.[2] Some of the most critical public health victories, such as reduced rates of smoking, lead poisoning, and motor vehicle-related deaths, along with increased life expectancy, are the direct result of policy and policy advocacy.

Public policy can address complex societal issues that drive health outcomes, such as affordable housing, improved safety and availability of all transportation modes, and access to education. To be effective in policy development, public health practitioners need to know how to identify and evaluate problems, isolate root causes, analyze the evidence, and develop viable policy solutions. This proven, formulaic approach to policy development is essential, albeit insufficient. More than anything, public health practitioners need to know how to tell a compelling story.

Comedian George Carlin once observed of homelessness:

> I'll tell you what they ought to do about homelessness. First thing: Change the name of it. Change the name of the condition. It's not homelessness; it's houselessness. It's houses these people need. A home is an abstract idea. A home is a setting, it's a state of mind. These people need houses—physical, tangible structures.[3]

This quote masterfully illustrates the importance of a narrative arc, which is the cornerstone of good policy development. Homelessness is a multifaceted concern that intersects multiple systems. Many people who experience homelessness need access to wraparound services and programs to support their mental and physical well-being; however, as the comedian points out, permanent, stable housing is the essential need of those experiencing homelessness. Framing the problem in this way positions housing as a solution.

Defining a problem is the first, and arguably the most significant, step in policy development because it dictates solutions. Further, it requires the ability to distinguish the symptoms or the effects of a problem from the actual underlying problem. Simply put, different definitions result in different solutions. For example, defining obesity as being a result of individual behavior (e.g., eating habits) leaves little room for a viable policy solution, because changes to individual behavior are not easy to legislate. If instead obesity is defined as an experience that results from economic and structural conditions, such as food access and costs, or lack of safe areas for exercise, systemic barriers are revealed for which legislation is a realistic remedy.

Failure to carefully define and then appropriately frame an issue allows the audience to deny or dismiss its impact—or worse, pretend that you are talking about something else entirely. How public health practitioners define and frame problems (e.g., purposefully illustrate the adverse conditions created by the problem) provides the audience with a particular mindset, and the power of a mindset is transformative as it shapes future thoughts, ideas, and actions. Translating complex data into a compelling story is one of the most significant ways public health practitioners can impact policy discussions and influence change.

Policy Engagement

Governmental public health practitioners should bear in mind that while policy advocacy may be a part of policy engagement, advocacy has a nuanced meaning. The World Health Organization defines advocacy as "a combination of individual and social actions designed to gain political commitment, policy support, social acceptance and systems support for a particular health goal or program."[4] Often, the goal of advocacy is to influence decision makers.

Engagement is typically a broader undertaking than advocacy, designed to inform and educate decision makers. The Centers for Disease Control and Prevention (CDC) defines stakeholder engagement as the process of identifying and connecting with "decision makers, partners, those affected by the policy, and the general public."[2] Given the complexity and limitations around what governmental public health practitioners can do in their capacity as government employees, this section focuses on the full spectrum of policy engagement, for practitioners as well as for interest groups. Understanding this process better positions public health practitioners for success.

Policy development and policy engagement are intertwined (figure 16.1). Policy engagement can take many forms depending on the audience or the advocate. In this chapter, the term *policy engagement* is defined as the process by which practitioners, advocates, organizations, business leaders, and others seek to elevate problems through education and advocacy, and influence policy decisions. Consider policy engagement across two domains: strategy and tactics.

Because governmental policy engagement seeks to inform and educate decision makers—typically elected officials—public health practitioners must have a keen understanding of the policymaking process and how government works. There is rarely a beginning or an end when it comes to the iterative and often messy process. This is especially true when political interests and motives are at play. Many political nuances may not be readily known to public health

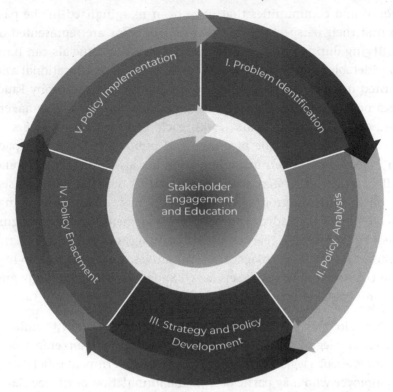

Figure 16.1. The policy development, enactment, and implementation process. Source: Redrawn from "CDC Policy Process," Centers for Disease Control and Prevention, May 29, 2015, https://www.cdc.gov/policy/polaris/policyprocess/index.html. Public domain.

practitioners; however, approaching policymaking with sensitivity and an eye toward solutions-oriented change helps to position real people and real issues, not politics, at the center of sustainable systemic change.

Policy engagement strategy requires assessing the political landscape, understanding the policymaking process, and evaluating where you are currently, where you want to go (your policy "ask"), and how you intend to get there (the tactics you will use). Policy engagement tactics are the specific actions and activities you will deploy to capture the attention of those you wish to inform and educate. Some tactics to consider include coalition-building with groups and communities that have been marginalized in the past so that their perspectives and real-life concerns are represented or testifying during public hearings. Governmental officials can have considerable impact behind the scenes, serving as educational and trusted resources to policymakers. For example, Dr. Anthony Fauci became a highly visible, respected health voice for policymakers because of his many years working closely with all members of Congress in one-on-one meetings and public forums. His impact far exceeded his governmental position because of his translational skills and direct, honest style. Additional tactics that may be used by outside interest groups, some of which may constitute lobbying, include grassroots advocacy, paid advertisements and campaigns, media advocacy (e.g., earned media coverage, op-eds, letters to the editor, and social media), ballot initiatives, and direct lobbying. The U.S. Internal Revenue Service (IRS) defines direct lobbying and grassroots lobbying as follows:

> Direct lobbying communication refers to any attempt to influence any legislation through communication with a member or employee of a legislative or similar body; a government official or employee who may participate in the formulation of the legislation; or the general public in a referendum, initiative, constitutional amendment, or similar procedure.
>
> Grassroots lobbying communication refers to any attempt to influence any legislation through an attempt to affect the opinions of the general public or any part of the general public.[5]

There are clear limitations to what governmental public health practitioners are allowed to do.[6] What is allowable depends on the funding source and the rules and empowerment of a practitioner's organization or department. In this chapter, the universe of policy engagement includes activities that may be impermissible for health practitioners in government. Whatever the tactic or tactics chosen, there are six keys to success when it comes to policy engagement: know your ask; know your audience, supporters, and decision makers; know and engage the opposition; develop consistent and clear messaging; consider timing; and stay the course.

Know Your Ask

After completing the hard work of identifying and assessing a problem, isolating the root causes, analyzing the evidence, and developing viable policy solutions, practitioners must know what they want and how they believe they can achieve it. An "ask" is more than the outcome. It must also include the process undertaken to reach the outcome. In other words, what is your specific policy objective and how do you envision realizing that objective? What do you seek— a budget allocation, introduction of legislation, regulatory change, increased issue awareness? Knowing your ask is the single most critical aspect of policy engagement, because everything else derives from it. Once you know exactly what you want and how you want to achieve it, you then need to assess who can deliver what you seek.

Know Your Audience (Supporters/Decision Makers)

Governmental policy engagement requires an analysis of those in power. Whom do you aim to convince—legislators or executive department administrators? What motivates the decision makers? Have they championed other issues that closely align with the policy change you seek? Answers to these questions will help practitioners home in on their core audience and determine how best to design messages that compel action—or at the very least resonate enough to spark interest and dialogue.

Knowing the audience also means identifying and analyzing stakeholders who can help to build an enabling environment for policy change. "There is power in numbers," Dr. Martin Luther King Jr. said. While a vocal mass helps to create power and amplifies collective voices to drive long-standing policy change, it is important to be thoughtful and strategic when identifying allies. Engaging others on a topic for the sake of driving up numbers does a disservice to your goals. You should identify and enlist those allies who (1) have a unique perspective or a shared stake in the issue, (2) possess close relationships with the decision makers you want to influence, (3) have access to an organized network around which to build a meaningful alliance, and/or (4) are credible and respected messengers whom the decision makers trust.

Finally, it is critical to know who is most impacted by your policy solution. Have they been engaged? Do they believe the policy solution you are advocating for is right for them? Too often, researchers, practitioners, advocates, and others make assumptions about what certain populations or communities want or need and craft solutions based on those assumptions. Make an earnest, deliberate, and continuous effort to get to know the constituency that your policy solution targets. Having their early support will further your path to successful engagement. Community participation is an ongoing process and ensures equitable outcomes by centering those most affected—giving them voice so that they see themselves reflected in the work—and allows them to be the architects of change.

Know and Engage the Opposition

A related aspect of knowing your audience is identifying those standing in your way. Who is opposed to your policy recommendation, and why? Do they have enough influence that your efforts could be derailed? Can they mobilize quickly? Are they open to compromise?

In the book *Making Research Evidence Matter: A Guide to Policy Advocacy in Transition Countries,*[7] the authors define policy advocacy: "Policy advocacy is the process of negotiating and mediating a dialogue through which influential networks, opinion leaders, and, ultimately, decision makers take ownership of your ideas, evidence, and proposals, and subsequently act upon them." This definition points up the importance of compromise through negotiation. Knowing your opposition helps you focus on the most salient aspects of your policy argument and prepares you to counter the opposing narrative. In addition, it allows you to discover any synergy that could propel a compromise. Define your audience (supporters and those opposed) early and engage them often. Never assume that perceived opponents are against your positions—often, they may have common interests and values that can be aligned with your efforts.

An example from 2010 is the modernization of the U.S. Food and Drug Administration (FDA) food inspection authorities. Traditionally, many viewed the food industry as a monolithic force opposed to increased government regulation. A coalition of public interest organizations, including consumer groups, food-borne illness victims, and public health associations, conducted extensive outreach and research into understanding the industry's position. As part of this analysis, food safety reform advocates recognized that large food corporations were concerned that broad recalls (which often misidentify the actual source) and high-profile food-related outbreaks were unnecessarily hurting their brands. Eventually, the association representing these brands, the Grocery Manufacturers Association, joined the public interest community to support the FDA Food Safety Modernization Act of 2011. That alliance of "odd bedfellows" tipped the scales, generating widespread bipartisan support for a policy that previously lacked political will.

Remember, policymaking is iterative, which leaves room to tweak your ask, double down on the tactics you use, and identify a path forward if opposition is unwilling to negotiate.

Develop Clear, Concise, and Consistent Messaging

In *Making Research Evidence Matter*, the authors explain:

> In presenting policy research to any audience, there is a tendency for those from a research or academic background to place too much emphasis on the research process itself and the details of the experiment. Audiences interested in public policy problems tend to be of mixed backgrounds, and normally have limited interest in or capacity to absorb the details of your research; what really interests them is the implications of your findings for the current policy challenges and discussion.[7]

Policymakers deal with hundreds of different issues at any single moment, from constituent requests for pothole repair, concerns about crime spikes, and requests to review and approve new development deals to calls for program funding and impactful new legislation. Given the competing demands on their time, you need to craft messages that are memorable and get to the point. Through your extensive research and analysis, you likely will have generated copious evidence, reflections, and findings. Resist the urge to go in-depth in your messaging and instead distill down to the takeaway messages. If the decision makers have only a few moments to hear your argument, what is your pitch? What is the most important message for them to walk away with? All of your communications should clearly, consistently, and concisely articulate the policy problem, why it matters, and the solution and its impacts. Your goal is to convince decision makers to take a different position. As discussed above, the power of a mindset is transformative as it shapes future thoughts, ideas, and actions.

Timing Is Everything

Elected officials have a finite period while in office for effecting change. For this reason, they make decisions and take action on some policy issues and ignore others, whether intentionally or by circumstance. These priorities form the basis of a governmental policy agenda. Understanding which issues are top of mind for decision makers helps you determine whether there is a call for change and gauge momentum. As Dr. Martin Luther King Jr. said, there is power in numbers, and it is far easier to advance policy when there is a call for action from the public, advocates, and others engaged on a particular topic. If the issue is already on the agenda for policymakers, the time is ripe to act.

You have the best chance of influencing policy change when your evidence, research, and solutions are ready to feed into a policy discussion at, or just before, the time a policy decision is made. Part of the policy engagement strategy requires an understanding of the political landscape and the policymaking process. This information helps you to plan, prepare, predict, and participate in the ever-changing windows of opportunity that open and close during policymaking.

Stay the Course

"What Is Dead May Never Die," an episode title from the HBO series *Game of Thrones*, conveys a sentiment that rings true in the policy world. There are few truly novel issues; even if you are unsuccessful in your effort to socialize a specific policy and engage in the broader policy discussion, topics you are passionate about will re-emerge.

You will have your day in the sun. Not every failed attempt means the effort was a failure; sometimes the battle to effect long-standing policy change is won incrementally. The first engagement may not have yielded the outcome you hoped for, but it unquestionably raised awareness and centered the problem and your solution in the public's consciousness. Future engagement will be much easier, because educating decision makers or the public will require fewer resources and less time.

Policy Action in Practice: A Case Study

Kansas City, Missouri, is a growing and dynamic midwestern city, which like many urban municipalities has demonstrated a widespread commitment to high-quality prekindergarten (pre-K). Leaders in the community, government, and businesses agreed that the Kansas City region needed to expand access to excellent pre-K. In 2019, residents were asked to vote on a ballot initiative to raise the city's sales tax to boost local education programs, equipment, and teachers for four- and five-year-olds. With 67% of voters voting no, the ballot initiative failed.

To understand how a policy that garnered universal support ultimately failed, you must understand the landscape and context in which the issue arose. Here is an analysis of lessons learned in Kansas City.

ISSUE

The need for improved access to quality pre-K was evidenced by the fact that only 34% of Kansas City's four-year-olds attended a quality pre-K program, and only 33% of children in Kansas City could read at grade level by the end of third grade. In April 2019, the Pre-K for KC initiative appeared on the ballot. Question 1 asked voters to support a plan to raise the Kansas City sales tax by three-eighths of a cent for a 10-year period, generating an estimated $30 million per year. Funds would be used to provide access to year-round educational opportunities for four- and five-year-olds before they entered kindergarten. The initiative failed, with two-thirds of voters rejecting Question 1.

BACKGROUND/CONTEXT

There are more than 15 public school districts that are either wholly or partially located in Kansas City, Missouri, as well as more than 20 public charter schools. The city government does not have formal jurisdiction over any of them. Recognizing the need for, and importance of, increasing school readiness, Kansas City's mayor released a plan to improve access to high-quality pre-K across the city. In developing the plan, the mayor consulted with business leaders, subject matter experts, education professionals, and others. To elevate the issue and increase support, the business and civic community ran a public campaign focused on building citywide awareness of the importance of early childhood education. Specifically, the campaign discussed the benefits of early childhood education to children's kindergarten readiness and academic success, rather than the details of the plan or its funding approach.

OPPOSITION

Despite the mayor's efforts, all school districts within city limits, with the exception of the charter schools, opposed the plan. Reasons for opposition were myriad. Many parties believed the mayor's office did not do enough to engage all stakeholders; consultations with school superintendents did not begin until two months before the plan was released. Additionally, the school districts had three main objections to the plan: First, opponents believed the plan would provide public funds to private schools or religious schools, which they considered a voucher program. Second, they believed that under the plan there would be no role for school boards. The initiative proposed one plan and imposed it on all school districts, regardless of their approach to pre-K. Finally, the opposition disagreed with the implementation structure, which they viewed as bureaucratic and shifting power to entities outside the education sector. There also was strong disagreement about funding. Opponents felt a sales tax was the wrong approach because it would use economic development funds for pre-K, and many people believed those funds should be used for other priorities. The civil rights community viewed the sales tax as a regressive approach that disproportionately shifted costs.

For these reasons, opponents mobilized and ran their own campaign, with messaging focused on support for universal pre-K and opposition to the mayor's specific approach. They identified a different funding mechanism, a property tax increase, to support pre-K expansion—an effort that was under way before the mayor's plan was launched. Opponents had a big win the week before the vote, when the *Kansas City Star* published an editorial recommending that readers vote No on Question 1. The editorial board said the plan was too expensive, had a confusing structure, used a regressive sales tax for its funding mechanism, and was opposed by the city's educators and community groups.

LESSONS LEARNED

After specifics of the mayor's plan were released, strong opposition surfaced. While supporters and opponents agreed on the need for quality pre-K, they disagreed on the funding mechanism and overall approach. Below, we apply the six keys for successful policy engagement to the Kansas City example.

Know Your Ask

Knowing your ask is about what you want and how you want to achieve it. Everyone, including the initiative's opponents, agreed that the city needed to expand access to high-quality pre-K programs, but there was disagreement about the process for achieving that objective. The universality of support for pre-K likely led supporters of Question 1 to believe that the "how" of improving school readiness—through imposition of a sales tax—was inconsequential. That assumption dealt a blow that helped the initiative to fail.

Knowing exactly what you want and how you want to achieve it is the critical first step of policy engagement; everything else follows.

Know Your Audience

A vital aspect of knowing your audience is understanding who will be most impacted by your policy solutions/objectives and ensuring that you are actively and deliberately engaging those audiences early and often. In Kansas City, business leaders, community groups, school administrators, and government alike recognized the urgent need to support the city's earliest learners by increasing access to quality pre-K programs. Critical segments of those supporters, however—school administrators and educators—were not engaged until after the plan was developed. Because the mayor's team did not consult with school superintendents until two months before the plan was made public, stakeholders could not meaningfully help shape what the plan could become. As a result, would-be supporters dissented and launched their own campaign, which stalled the shared goal of seeing pre-K enhanced, because Question 1 was defeated.

Know and Engage the Opposition

In Kansas City, the audience for improving pre-K was vast, consisting of the public, superintendents, schoolteachers, students, and the business community. Universally, there was support for expanded pre-K, but the method chosen to fund this effort proved divisive. Part of knowing your audience and engaging your opposition is the opportunity to assess synergy and to negotiate. Bring together those who agree with your position and those who oppose it throughout the process to find a common goal. Collaboration with stakeholders (those in support of your effort and those opposed) should begin at the nascent stage, not after the decision makers have met and developed a plan. This negotiation/collaboration must commence in order to reach an agreement about both the problem and the solution. While they may be tedious, community participation and stakeholder engagement are necessities. The process must be ongoing to ensure equitable outcomes by centering those most impacted, giving them voice so that they see themselves reflected in the work.

As already described, it is important to understand whom your policy proposal or recommendation will most impact. In Kansas City, since jurisdiction over education rested with the school superintendents, the public deferred to their views, making the superintendents' opposition especially detrimental. The superintendents had significant influence in their communities and having their buy-in early on would likely have changed the outcome. Be mindful as you develop your strategy and think through the tactics you will deploy if you are unable to garner the support of a critical mass of influencers; you need to be creative and nimble enough to switch your approach to account for the opposition.

As we have noted, nuanced political realities can be unknown to public health practitioners. Nevertheless, practitioners must approach the policymaking process with sensitivity and an understanding of the stakeholders involved, the climate in a particular jurisdiction, and an appreciation for work that may already have been done on a specific topic. A regional approach, like the one proposed in Kansas City, countered local positions and differences and ignored what was already happening around the area regarding pre-K. This led to rejection of the ballot initiative.

Develop Clear, Concise, and Consistent Messaging

Campaign messaging should address opponents and explain why other policy options are not viable. In Kansas City, the campaign messaging focused almost exclusively on the benefits of pre-K without ever discussing specifics of the plan. Once details of the plan emerged, opponents developed strategic messaging that simultaneously acknowledged and supported the benefits of pre-K and condemned the mayor's funding mechanism. They presented an alternative funding proposal, suggesting that voters consider a different funding option for achieving the same common goal. Supporters' messaging never addressed the opponents' position, making the case for the initiative less compelling. The editorial board of the *Kansas City Star* found opponents' arguments persuasive and recommended that readers vote No on Question 1.

Timing Is Everything

At the outset of policy engagement, make sure to understand the political climate and broader policy landscape, because these factors may compel a shift in timing. In the Kansas City case, at the time the mayor's plan was proposed, seven city council members were on the ballot to replace the mayor and thus had their own politics and priorities to manage. Also, before the ballot initiative launched, school superintendents were working on their own proposals to address pre-K. Timing of the funding ask also mattered: In 2019, there was a significant level of "tax fatigue" in Kansas City. The mayor's office had run 18 different tax campaigns and won 16 of them; that context helped make an additional sales tax proposal untenable.

Stay the Course

Even if you lose the battle, you may not lose the war. There may be wins in educating the public on the benefits of a specific policy solution or recommendation for future campaigns. In Kansas City, many supporters of the policy objective acknowledged that they spent nearly half a million dollars on the effort to expand Pre-K and lost, but they remained hopeful because they brought attention to the subject and felt strongly that they were on the right side of the issue. The more your issues are publicly discussed and debated, the greater the chance a city, state, or even the federal government will take action to adopt your policy solutions.

Conclusion

Some of the nation's greatest public health successes would not have been realized without policy change. The CDC's list of the "Ten Great Public Health Achievements"—including motor vehicle safety, tobacco control, and maternal and infant health—all involved policy change.[8] Public health practitioners are uniquely positioned to influence and impact policy change through strong policy development, compelling storytelling, and effective policy engagement. Utilizing the skills just discussed, public health professionals can champion evidence-based, expertise-based, and experience-based policy solutions to ensure that all people, regardless of race, religion, gender identity/expression, sexual orientation, education, or zip code, can live their healthiest possible life.

References

1. Institute of Medicine (US) Committee on Assuring the Health of the Public in the 21st Century, *The Future of the Public's Health in the 21st Century* (Washington, DC: National Academies Press, 2002), https://www.ncbi.nlm.nih.gov/books/NBK221239/.
2. "CDC Policy Process," Centers for Disease Control and Prevention, May 29, 2015, https://www.cdc.gov/policy/polaris/policyprocess/index.html.

3. George Carlin, "A War on Homelessness," from *Jammin in New York* (HBO, 1992), https://www.youtube.com/watch?v=lncLOEqc9Rw&t=246s.

4. Division of Health Education et al., *Advocacy Strategies for Health Development: Development Communication in Action* (Geneva, Switzerland: WHO, 1992), https://apps.who.int/iris/bitstream/handle/10665/70051/HED_92.4_eng.pdf.

5. Internal Revenue Service, "Instructions for Schedule C (Form 990) (2021)," https://www.irs.gov/instructions/i990sc.

6. *Anti-Lobbying Restrictions for CDC Grantees*, Centers for Disease Control and Prevention, April 2017, https://www.cdc.gov/grants/documents/Anti-Lobbying-Restrictions.pdf.

7. Eon Young and Lisa Quinn, *Making Research Evidence Matter: A Guide to Policy Advocacy in Transition Countries* (Budapest, Hungary: Open Society Foundations, 2012), https://advocacyguide.icpolicyadvocacy.org/sites/icpa-book.local/files/Policy_Advocacy_Guidebook_2012.pdf.

8. Keshia M. Pollack Porter, Lainey Rutkow, and Emma E. McGinty, "The Importance of Policy Change for Addressing Public Health Problems," *Sage Journals* 33, no. 1 (2018): 9–14, https://journals.sagepub.com/doi/full/10.1177/0033354918788880.

Evidence-Based Policymaking and Public Health Practice

MARCUS PLESCIA AND ROSS C. BROWNSON

DURING THE 1960S, OVER HALF the U.S. adult population smoked. Cigarettes were effectively marketed as safe, sophisticated, and sexy. Advertisements featured physicians pitching their favorite, "less irritating" brands. But public health professionals started to question cigarette safety as evidence began to mount that smoking had an increasing number of deleterious health effects. The evidence culminated in the 1964 U.S. Surgeon General's report on smoking, which launched one of the most successful public health efforts in recent times.[1]

As evidence grew, investigators determined that most adults started smoking as children and that widespread educational interventions were not effective. The public health approach shifted to policy interventions. Banning smoking in closed spaces, such as airplane cabins, and taxing products to make them more expensive, limiting advertising, and raising the age of purchase were all proven effective, especially with youth. Over time, smoking bans expanded to other indoor areas and work sites to limit secondhand exposure, and

Marcus Plescia and Ross C. Brownson, *Evidence-Based Policymaking and Public Health Practice*
In: *Building Strategic Skills for Better Health: A Primer for Public Health Professionals*. Edited by: Michael
R. Fraser and Brian C. Castrucci, Oxford University Press. © de Beaumont Foundation 2024.
DOI: 10.1093/oso/9780197744604.003.0018

ultimately changed social norms and acceptance of smoking. Recent policies have banned flavored tobacco products, regulated Internet sales, increased the age of purchase to 21, and limited retail sales. National smoking rates are now around 10%, a four-fifths decrease brought about by sustained evidence-based policy interventions at the local, state, and federal levels.

Few public health professionals would dispute the importance of evidence-based practice. Significant improvements in public health can be credited to the successful implementation of scientifically driven interventions that have proven population impact. Over the last two decades, public health has made considerable progress in developing the evidence base and learning how best to disseminate interventions. Effective sanitation practices, control of infectious diseases through immunization, changes in product design to reduce injuries, and discouragement of risky behaviors like tobacco use are all examples of successful evidence-based public health practice.

Evidence-based practice has been embraced in many health-related disciplines, and much can be learned from the experience in clinical medicine.

While significant challenges and undesired practices remain, development over the last 20 years of a well-developed culture and norm of evidence-based medical practice has helped balance traditional reliance on clinical experience with evidence from clinical research. Evidence-based practice is now the core of medical training both in the classroom and at the bedside. As a result, medical practices have ready access to the scientific literature to learn from the evidence, and information systems, such as electronic health records, have been tailored and improved to prompt evidence-based action and access to practice guidelines.

The practice of evidence-based public health faces both challenges and opportunities not applicable to medical practice. Public health studies are inherently more heterogeneous and more difficult to design. They frequently rely on interpretation of natural experiments and may involve multiple blended interventions in a community of diverse and often disparate groups. While they are challenging to study and evaluate, public health approaches allow creativity that ultimately makes their application in community settings more relevant and productive.

This chapter describes specific resources and steps to help public health practitioners (1) identify evidence-based policies and practices, (2) access and understand policy interventions that are promising or emerging, and (3) develop and implement sound public health policies and regulations. The chapter focuses primarily on "big P" policies (i.e., laws and administrative regulations) as opposed to "little p" policies (i.e., organizational policies and professional guidelines), although many of the same principles apply to either type of policy translation.

Evidence-Based Public Health Policy

Public health policies and regulatory actions are the foundation of strategies that focus on improving health across communities and populations. They are important because they affect large numbers of people, often require far fewer resources than more labor-intensive individual interventions, and are more likely to be sustained. They have been used to reduce infectious disease outbreaks, improve sanitation, and limit exposure to health risks in the environment. Requiring restaurants to comply with regular sanitation inspections and requiring youth vaccinations for school enrollment are important and effective examples that have been in place for decades. Recently, policies have been used to discourage risky health practices like smoking and to remove barriers to healthy behaviors like good nutrition and regular physical activity. These approaches are intended to "make the healthy choice the easy choice" and are particularly effective in communities that have limited resources and public investment. For example, multiuse policies in public school systems make physical activity resources like playing fields and walking and running tracks accessible to local communities on weekends or after hours.

The importance, urgency, and challenges of evidence-based public health policy interventions have been particularly relevant in the response to the COVID-19 pandemic. The evidence on effective policy interventions to control the spread of this infection evolved over the course of the pandemic response. Regulations like mandated use of masks, gathering restrictions, and stay-at-home/shelter-in-place orders were proven effective at limiting exposure and reducing rates of infection.[2-4] However, they also had uneven support and messaging from policy leaders, resulting in widespread public controversy and highly variable enactment among states and communities—often resulting in the undermining of public health powers.

Identifying Evidence-Based Practices and Policies

Evidence-based public health has been defined as "the process of integrating science-based interventions with community preferences to improve the health of populations."[5] Key components of evidence-based public health include making decisions based on the best available, peer-reviewed evidence; using data and information systems rigorously; applying program planning frameworks; engaging the community in decision-making; conducting sound evaluations; and disseminating what is learned.[6]

Several resources to help identify evidence-based practices are easily available to public health practitioners. For example, the Agency for Healthcare Research and Quality supports the *Guide to Clinical Preventive Services* (also known as the Clinical Guide), which is maintained by a panel of independent scientists and experts.[7] This text has a substantial impact on policy because it sets the standard for the clinical public health interventions that the Affordable Care Act mandates as reimbursable services. A population-based companion is *The Guide to Community Preventive Services* (the Community Guide), supported by the Centers for Disease Control and Prevention (CDC), which also is maintained by a panel of experts and identifies evidence-based interventions for population-based applications.[8] The Community Guide is easily navigable; it has an active web interface with the practice community and publicizes new recommendations through national organizations, funders, and social media. Unlike the Clinical Guide, however, the Community Guide is not used to set policy for reimbursable programs or services.

Other well-developed clinical evidence reviews like the Cochrane Library provide evidence-based recommendations for clinical preventive services and some community-based interventions.[9] Healthy People 2030 resources are an accessible source of objectives based on evidence-based practice. *What Works for Health*,[10] National Cancer Institute's Evidence-Based Cancer Control Programs (EBCCP),[11] CDC's *HIV Prevention that Works*,[12] and the Office of Adolescent Health's *Evidence-based Teen Pregnancy Prevention Programs*[13] are examples of several reputable sources of evidence-based practice for specific public health issues. These resources and others are widely available to public health practitioners and should be their first stop in promoting, developing, and designing community-based interventions.

The Clinical Guide and resources that define evidence-based practice have limited capacity to provide exhaustive and timely review and categorization of all emerging public health science. In addition, some recommendations identify science that is promising but that does not meet the exacting standards for evidence-based practice. As a result, the public health workforce must be able to access and interpret basic information from the scientific literature and apply it to practice.

Gaining access to published studies in peer-reviewed journals can be tedious and frustrating for even the most determined public health practitioner. The general lack of access to digital library resources is a significant challenge for many working in applied public health settings. At present, only 28% of scholarly publications can be accessed for free over the Internet,[14] and the remainder are controlled by publishing companies that charge user fees. Digital libraries at medical schools or large health sciences university programs are the most robust and comprehensive source of scientific publications, but their agreements with publishers limit use to students and faculty. Health department staff with faculty positions in public health schools may have some access to these digital libraries, but sharing this access with colleagues is formally prohibited.

Recently, the National Library of Medicine developed a program to allow state health departments to access a curated collection of scientific journals and other resources for a relatively modest fee.[15] Negotiating a process for interlibrary loans from a local library partner makes available journals that are not in the collection, and a modest budget can support purchase of others. Currently, about half of state health departments participate in this service.

Challenges of Evidence-Based Policymaking

Sources like the Community Guide and the Cochrane and Campbell review libraries have found enough evidence to designate a significant number of major legal interventions effective.[16] However, while public health policies can be highly effective and far-reaching, they also can have unintended consequences. When making and introducing public health policy, practitioners should exercise caution if impact, effectiveness, and potential unintended consequences are not known. Prohibition laws in the early 20th century were intended to reduce alcoholism and family violence. While rates of alcohol-related liver disease declined during Prohibition, it was ultimately repealed because the laws were hard to enforce and were associated with significant increases in organized crime. Today's policies to reduce significant increases in prescription opioid use through stronger prescribing regulations are considered by some to have led to an increase in use of heroin and other more potent illicit drugs.

State and local governments are known as the laboratories of democracy because most federal legislation originates from successful state and local laws. However, the process of crafting public policy is often compared to the process of making sausage—best not to watch it being made. While the use of evidence-based policy is desirable, it is sensitive to the political process, and proven practices may be hard to replicate across different communities. In addition, political leaders often need to act on high-profile health issues when evidence about effectiveness is not available. In Canada and Australia, the term *evidence-informed decision-making* is commonly used.[16] The term was developed in part to emphasize that public health policy decisions are based on research but also require consideration of political and organizational factors, such as politics, habits and traditions, pragmatics, resources, values, and ethics.[17,18]

At times, political ideology may be contrary to what science recommends. Water fluoridation programs are safe and highly effective in preventing dental disease, but they have been overturned in several communities. Industries like tobacco, sugar, and alcohol may oppose policies that are not in their interest by removing integral language or diminishing enforcement mechanisms. The tobacco industry has increasingly worked to pass less effective tobacco-use policies statewide and then has inserted "preemptive" language that limits the ability of communities to pass stronger, more effective policies at the local level. The vaping/electronic cigarette industry has used harm-reduction arguments to justify their products and to limit regulation, but the products' popularity and increasing use by youth have been alarming, and an outbreak of related lung injuries finally precipitated more substantive regulatory policies.

Policymaking in Emerging Situations

During most of the COVID-19 pandemic, state and local governments led the response to mitigate and control the rate of infection. Many states enacted policies and regulations at the state and municipality levels that protected much of the population during the early stages of the pandemic.[19] Often, local public health jurisdictions took earlier action and/or enacted more extensive regulations than the state to require use of face coverings in public settings, to restrict social gatherings, and to limit exposure through stay-at-home orders. The process was highly politicized and varied across regions, however, with Republican leaders slower to implement these policies during the most critical periods.[20]

In addition, identifying, defining, and implementing evidence-based policy interventions in a rapidly expanding pandemic were challenging for public health practitioners. Early on, respected scientific establishments like the CDC delayed guidance supporting the use of face masks because there was limited understanding of effectiveness. Many leaders, including the U.S. Surgeon General, initially urged the public to refrain from wearing N-95 or surgical masks, which were in short supply for healthcare workers. They then reversed course and instructed the public to wear cloth face masks in public settings and encouraged public mandates. This led to significant derision, confusion, and mistrust that undermined the public's trust in other regulations.

In many instances, action is needed before evidence about benefits or harms of policies and regulations is clear. Early in the pandemic, localities made the decision to close schools while the evidence of benefits or harms of closure was still emerging. School closure is a conventional infection-control policy and is frequently used during severe influenza outbreaks. It is also extremely disruptive and harmful to the growth and development of children, particularly those in situations where support and resources for virtual learning are limited. COVID-19 is rarely severe in children, and social distancing in school settings now appears to have been effective in limiting infection spread. Ultimately, the experience of reopening schools and the measures taken to reduce infection spread will inform future recommendations and policy.

Policy decisions about legalizing medicinal or recreational use of marijuana have been similarly challenging. Marijuana use is widespread in our society, but the legal consequences of sales or possession are unevenly applied and can be substantial. Furthermore, the potential health effects of regular and chronic marijuana use remain unclear. In the case of electronic cigarettes, which provide an inhaled form of nicotine without the dangerous byproducts of burning tobacco, the devices were heralded as less harmful than smoking and as a potential smoking cessation aid. Amid a lax regulatory response, accurate and consistent information about the ingredients and strength of the products was not available and use skyrocketed, particularly among youth who were not previous smokers. Ultimately, a likely contaminant led to multiple cases of severe lung damage and both state and federal policy efforts intensified to regulate electronic cigarettes and enforce current restrictions.

Authority versus Influence in Developing Public Health Policy

Many policies that can affect public health are not specific to the work, setting, or authority of public health agencies. For example, school nutrition and physical activity standards are important policy interventions to prevent childhood obesity, but state health officials do not have authority over separate state or local school agencies.

In other examples, organizations outside government, from private schools to major corporations, create work and facilities rules on matters as diverse as tobacco use and paid sick leave, and healthcare systems and insurers set coverage and payment policies that can be highly effective and far-reaching. Developing policy change in these areas of public health requires practitioners to use professional influence and boundary-spanning leadership skills to leverage relationships with leaders in other state agencies, Tribal communities, and healthcare and community settings.

CDC's 6|18 initiative outlines six high-burden health conditions and 18 interventions that are evidence-based, have potential for widespread impact, have acceptable costs and resource mechanisms, and are politically feasible.[21] The initiative provides a useful matrix for public health leaders seeking to prioritize the use of limited resources. New approaches, such as health impact assessments, which estimate the impact of a policy or intervention in non-health-related sectors—for example, agriculture, transportation, and economic development—help facilitate close collaboration with external agencies.[22]

Identifying and Monitoring Public Health Policies

Much of the work on public health policy at the state and local level is based on identifying, tracking, and at times evaluating what others have done to address a specific issue or health concern through laws or regulation. Often, this work is done by public health staff who do not have formal legal training. Policy surveillance—the ongoing, systematic collection, analysis, and dissemination of information about laws of health importance—is an important resource for public health staff. Policy surveillance reviews and technical assistance are available from groups like the CDC's Public Health Law Program, the Network for Public Health Law, the Public Health Law Center, the Public Health Advocacy Institute, and the Association of State and Territorial Health Officials, which compile and analyze policies on a range of specific issues. Groups like ChangeLab Solutions provide reviews and technical assistance while focusing on local laws and ordinances. More specialized data can be obtained for public health issues through groups like the Tobacco Control Legal Consortium, the Campaign for Tobacco Free Kids, and the Immunization Action Coalition.[23-25] The CDC also has policy subject matter focused on specific issues that can be easily identified by searching its website.

When organized policy reviews and analysis are not available, resources that provide scans and mapping of state public health laws may be useful. These include LawAtlas.org, which provides policy surveillance data sets and legal mapping tools on a variety of public health issues. The Prescription Drug Abuse Policy System (PDAPS), Alcohol Policy Information System, State Tobacco Activities Tracking and Evaluation System, and Americans for Nonsmokers' Rights (ANR) use similar platforms but are specific to substance misuse and alcohol and tobacco control-related policies. These platforms allow searches to be highly focused and link to actual text of a law.

When there is limited surveillance on a particular policy area, public health staff often do their own research. This requires specific training and some legal and subject matter expertise. The Policy Surveillance Program at Temple University's Beasley School of Law provides in-person and online training on policy surveillance methods.[26] Online subscription services, such as FiscalNote and Westlaw, compile information about federal and state statutes and bills. These services offer a system for tracking and categorizing legislation that was introduced, passed, or failed and often provide data for the preceding 10 years. Special interest groups that oppose public health efforts can be excellent sources of policy data and can provide insight to policy options that run counter to public health. Cannabis-use supporters and vaccine resistance groups, for example, often track legislation and compile results, which public health groups can themselves use to monitor policy activity.

Communicating Evidence-Based Approaches to Policymakers

To effectively communicate evidence-based approaches to policymakers, research and data supporting the policy actions must be made available and accessible. Research findings and data are most effective when they (1) clearly identify a public health issue that should take priority over other issues, (2) demonstrate that there are interventions that will have significant impact, (3) can be applied to the local level and provide a compelling illustration of how lives are affected, and (4) estimate the cost of the intervention.[27]

While quantitative data are a powerful representation of scientific work, aggregated numbers and statistics like percentages or rates are not effective when policymakers have limited experience with data analysis and interpretation. Stories, on the other hand, are compelling to policymakers and to the political process. Adapting the inherently analytical and quantitative aspect of scientific research to this format can be challenging; take care to avoid making scientific findings that are objective and disciplined appear subjective or sensational. A story can show how a health issue affects individuals or a community and can reveal circumstances and barriers that limit or contribute to health and that can only be influenced by policy.

Stories can be especially useful in the case of a behavior change intervention by illustrating that it is not easy for some individuals to make healthy choices. For example, nutrition and physical activity changes are often more challenging for people in neighborhoods with limited grocery store options and restricted access to recreation. Communicating with policymakers requires a concise format that minimizes professional jargon and analytics. It must demonstrate the need to act, describe specific policy interventions, and explain why they will be effective. Policy briefs are frequently used for this purpose. Several essential elements of a good policy brief are:[28]

1. An informative title that motivates the audience to read on.
2. A compelling narrative or story.
3. Discussion of the scale/importance of the problem using epidemiology in a format that is easy to understand and provides context (e.g., the number of Americans who died of opioid overdoses in 2018, which is greater than the number who died in the Vietnam war). It may be effective to highlight certain populations (e.g., racial/ethnic minorities) who are experiencing health disparities.

4. Explanation of the benefits of intervention with a focus on public health prevention and the impact (e.g., the number of overdoses that could be prevented if naloxone, which can reverse an overdose, were available as over-the-counter treatment).

5. Overview of the evidence-based policy options. Refer to summaries of the literature, such as systematic reviews or similar authoritative sources (e.g., the Community Guide), as well as data on cost-effectiveness, when available.

6. Policy recommendation. Whether to provide a policy recommendation or to remain neutral or nonpartisan depends on the author's perception of the audience as well as the author's role in the process.

7. Sources consulted or recommended. Legislators and their staff often use a policy brief as an introduction to the scientific sources and websites where they can learn more.

Implementing and Evaluating Public Health Policies

New policies must be communicated effectively, and a notification period can help prepare the public for significant change. Engaging communities through approaches like community-based participatory research and community-oriented primary care provides valuable insight into cultural and historical perspectives and builds trust that may ultimately allow greater cooperation and more equitable participation.

Policies that help set new social norms may find success because of social expectations and peer pressure. However, most policies require some form of enforcement and consequences. These components should be built into policies with procedures for monitoring compliance and assessing reasonable penalties for violations, as well as clear descriptions of to whom the policy applies and who is accountable for enforcement. In addition, public health policy often must be enacted with other policies or social interventions that support and facilitate compliance. The COVID-19 pandemic taught us how hard it is to enact successful quarantine and isolation interventions without unemployment support, access to housing, food security, and other wraparound services.

Evaluation of public health policy interventions is a process that should be built into all public health efforts.[6] Compelling public health issues often capture the attention of the media and result in public demand for action. If evidence-based interventions have not been developed, policymakers may experiment with approaches based on intuition, personal experience, or dogma. These approaches should be examined to determine if they are effective and to ensure that they do not result in unanticipated harms. In addition, as policies are tested and new research is conducted, laws should be amended to reflect the available science. Child safety-seat laws, for example, have changed many times over the years to reflect new evidence, technology, and standards.[16]

Summary

Better integration of the science and practice of applied public health will result in more effective and appropriate policy interventions in states and communities across the nation. There are many resources available to the public health workforce for identifying evidence-based policy interventions and for monitoring policies enacted at the federal, state, and local levels. This information must be communicated effectively to policymakers and their staff. The political process makes the strict practice of enacting only evidence-based policies unrealistic, but public health can work to make policies as evidence-informed as possible and to advocate for strong evaluation plans to be included with innovative approaches that are yet to be fully assessed.

References
1. United States Public Health Service, Surgeon General's Report, *Smoking and Health: Report of the Advisory Committee to the Surgeon General of the Public Health Service* (Washington, DC: U.S. Department of Health, Education, and Welfare, 1964).
2. Miriam E. Van Dyke et al., "Trends in County-Level COVID-19 Incidence in Counties with and without a Mask Mandate—Kansas, June

1–August 23, 2020," *Morbidity and Mortality Weekly Report* 69, no. 47 (2020): 1777–1781, https://www.cdc.gov/mmwr/volumes/69/wr/mm694 7e2.htm.

3. Florence A. Kanu et al., "Declines in SARS-CoV-2 Transmission, Hospitalizations, and Mortality after Implementation of Mitigation Measures—Delaware, March–June 2020," *Morbidity and Mortality Weekly Report* 69, no. 45 (2020): 1691–1694, https://www.cdc.gov/mmwr/volu mes/69/wr/mm6945e1.htm.

4. M. Shayne Gallaway et al., "Trends in COVID-19 Incidence after Implementation of Mitigation Measures—Arizona, January 22–August 7, 2020," *Morbidity and Mortality Weekly Report* 69, no.40 (2020), 1460–1463, https://www.cdc.gov/mmwr/volumes/69/wr/mm6940e3.htm.

5. Neal D. Kohatsu, Jennifer G. Robinson, and James C. Torner, "Evidence-Based Public Health: An Evolving Concept," *American Journal of Preventative Medicine* 27, no. 5 (2004): 417–428, https://pubmed.ncbi. nlm.nih.gov/15556743/.

6. Ross C. Brownson, Jonathan E. Fielding, and Christopher M. Maylahn, "Evidence-Based Public Health: A Fundamental Concept for Public Health Practice," *Annual Review of Public Health* 30, (2009): 175–201, https://pubmed.ncbi.nlm.nih.gov/19296775/.

7. U.S. Preventive Services Task Force, *The Guide to Clinical Preventive Services* https://www.uspreventiveservicestaskforce.org/Page/Name/ home.

8. *The Guide to Community Preventive Services*, https://www.thecommuni tyguide.org/.

9. *Cochrane Database of Systematic Reviews*, Cochrane Library, https://www. cochranelibrary.com/cdsr/about-cdsr.

10. *What Works for Health*, U.S. County Health Rankings, https://www. countyhealthrankings.org/take-action-to-improve-health/what-works-for-health.

11. The National Cancer Institute's Evidence-Based Cancer Control Programs (EBCCP), https://cancercontrolplanet.cancer.gov/planet/.

12. "Effective Interventions," Centers for Disease Control and Prevention, https://effectiveinterventions.cdc.gov/.

13. "Adolescent Health," Office of Adolescent Health, https://www.hhs.gov/ ash/oah/grant-programs/teen-pregnancy-prevention-program-tpp/ index.html.

14. Heather Piwowar et al., "The State of OA: A Large-Scale Analysis of the Prevalence and Impact of Open Access Articles." *PeerJ* 6 (2018): e4375, https://peerj.com/articles/4375/.

15. "About PHDL Collection," National Library of Medicine, https://old. nnlm.gov/nphco/collection.

16. Scott Burris et al., "Better Health Faster: The 5 Essential Public Health Law Services," *Public Health Reports* 131, no. 6 (2016): 747–753, https://pubmed.ncbi.nlm.nih.gov/28123219/.

17. Rebecca Armstrong, Tahna Pettman, and Elizabeth B. Waters, "Shifting Sands—From Descriptions to Solutions," *Public Health* 128, no. 6 (2014): 525–532, https://pubmed.ncbi.nlm.nih.gov/24916424/.

18. Sarah M. Viehbeck, Mark Petticrew, and Steven Cummins, "Old Myths, New Myths: Challenging Myths in Public Health," *American Journal of Public Health* 105, no. 4 (2015): 665–669, https://www.ncbi.nlm.nih.gov/pmc/articles/PMC4358183/.

19. Michael R. Fraser, Chrissie Juliano, and Gabrielle Nichols, "Variation among Public Health Interventions in Initial Efforts to Prevent the Control and Spread of COVID-19 in the 50 States, 29 Big Cities and the District of Columbia," *Journal of Public Health Management and Practice* 27, suppl. 1 (2021): S29–S38, https://pubmed.ncbi.nlm.nih.gov/33239561/.

20. Christopher Adolph et al., "Pandemic Politics: Timing of State-Level Social Distancing Responses to COVID-19," *Journal of Health Politics, Policy and Law* 46, no 2. (2021): 211–233, https://pubmed.ncbi.nlm.nih.gov/32955556/.

21. "CDC's 6|18 Initiative: Accelerating Evidence into Action," Centers for Disease Control and Prevention, October 4, 2018, https://www.cdc.gov/sixeighteen/index.html.

22. Karen Lock, "Health Impact Assessment," *BMJ* 320, no. 7246 (2000): 1395–1398, https://www.ncbi.nlm.nih.gov/pmc/articles/PMC1118057/.

23. Tobacco Control Laws, https://www.tobaccocontrollaws.org/.

24. "U.S. Initiatives," Campaign for Tobacco Free Kids, https://www.tobaccofreekids.org/what-we-do/us.

25. "State Laws and Mandates by Vaccine," Immunization Action Coalition, https://www.immunize.org/laws/.

26. Temple University Center for Public Health Law Research, http://publichealthlawresearch.org/

27. Thomas R. Frieden, "Six Components Necessary for Effective Public Health Program Implementation," *American Journal of Public Health* 104, no. 1 (2014): 17–22, https://www.ncbi.nlm.nih.gov/pmc/articles/PMC3910052/.

28. Katherine A. Stamatakis, Timothy D. McBride, and Ross C. Brownson, "Communicating Prevention Messages to Policy Makers: The Role of Stories in Promoting Physical Activity," *Journal of Physical Activity and Health*, suppl. 1 (2010): S99–S107, https://pubmed.ncbi.nlm.nih.gov/20440020/.

18

STRATEGIC SKILL IN FOCUS:
▶ *Data-Driven Decision-Making*

Public Health Informatics, Big Data, Advanced Analytics, and Emerging Technology

WILLIAM J. KASSLER

PUBLIC HEALTH PRACTICE COMPRISES A complex and wide-ranging set of functions that are information-rich and heavily quantitative. Collection, analysis, interpretation, and dissemination of data underlie most public health services, such as diagnosis and assessment, program design and implementation, and program monitoring and evaluation. Examples include public health surveillance of infectious and noncommunicable diseases and community health needs assessment. Both involve sifting through large amounts of raw data to glean information and synthesize that information into actionable knowledge for achieving program and policy goals.

Widespread adoption of relatively recent technologies, such as electronic health records (EHRs), smartphones, wearable devices, and social media, has resulted in exponential growth of available data. The data are large, messy, and often unstructured; arise from multiple nontraditional sources; and often do not fit neatly into

William J. Kassler, *Public Health Informatics, Big Data, Advanced Analytics, and Emerging Technology*
In: *Building Strategic Skills for Better Health: A Primer for Public Health Professionals.* Edited by: Michael R. Fraser and Brian C. Castrucci, Oxford University Press. © de Beaumont Foundation 2024.
DOI: 10.1093/oso/9780197744604.003.0019

standard databases. This presents both opportunities and challenges to public health systems and to those who practice in those systems. Surveillance, a foundational activity in public health practice, is well suited for technological innovation. But public health's ability to transform new data sources into useful information requires increasingly more advanced technology and analytic techniques.

The promise of big data and advanced analytics is fueling the need for a more specialized workforce.[1] This chapter focuses on the concepts of big data, technology, and analytics, as well as the strategic workforce skills necessary to take advantage of the opportunities. (See table 18.1 for definitions of key terms and concepts.)

Table 18.1. Definitions of Key Terms and Concepts

Artificial intelligence (AI)	AI is the process of making computers more intelligent by teaching systems to mimic human decision-making. Augmented intelligence emphasizes applications that keep humans in the loop (supporting decision-making rather than replacing people). AI is a suite of technologies, including, but not limited to, natural language processing, computer vision, and various forms of machine learning.
Big data	Big data is the term applied to very large data sets beyond the ability of traditional databases to capture, manage, and process. Big data typically have one or more of the following attributes: high volume, high velocity, or high variety. These data are often complex and messy, so veracity can be a challenge.
Cloud computing	Cloud computing is the delivery of information technology services, such as data storage and analytic applications, over the Internet, hosted by computer servers located off-premises. Often called simply "the cloud."
Computer vision	Computer vision is a form of AI that enables computer systems to extract meaningful information from photographs, videos, or other images and to process visual input in ways that are similar to how humans see.
Data scientist	A data scientist is a practitioner of a new multidisciplinary field that evolved to tackle the complexities of big data. A data scientist uses statistical methods, modeling, and computer science to extract insight and business value from data.
Informatics	Informatics is an interdisciplinary endeavor that applies information technology to systems engineering. Informatics blends the technical aspects of information systems (i.e., information and computer sciences) with a management approach to data governance, privacy, design, and workflow.

Table 18.1. Continued

Information systems	Information systems are a set of resources both technical (hardware, software, infrastructure) and human (trained personnel) organized for the collection, processing, maintenance, use, and dissemination of information.
Internet of Things (IoT)	The Internet of Things refers to the connection of a variety of consumer devices (beyond computers and smartphones) to the Internet. This allows devices to receive and act on information and enables data from sensors embedded within devices (such as fitness trackers, medical devices, and household electronics) to be collected and aggregated.
Machine learning	Machine learning is a form of AI in which a computer system learns from data rather than through explicit programming. Machine learning involves developing an algorithm, training it on a data set to develop mathematical models of the data, and inputting new data into the model to generate an output. Deep learning is a specialized form of machine learning that is patterned after neural networks.
Natural language processing (NLP)	NLP is a form of AI that uses computational linguistics to decipher speech and text and to process language in ways that are similar to how humans communicate. NLP powers chatbots and virtual assistants and is the way computer systems ingest and "understand" information from written sources, such as notes, websites, and articles.
Predictive analytics/ Predictive modeling	Predictive analytics/predictive modeling involves modeling historical data to predict the likelihood of future outcomes. Machine learning applied to big data is particularly well suited to predictive modeling.

Big Data

Traditional types of data used in public health research and practice include clinical data from medical records and claims, laboratory analysis, survey data, and place-based data on environmental or community characteristics. Innovative technologies present new forms and sources of data, but at the cost of increased complexity.[2] For example, widespread adoption of EHRs has unlocked massive amounts of clinical data that were previously inaccessible via manual chart abstraction. The digital footprints from our online presence, search logs, and social media feeds can be rich sources of behavioral and health status information. A proliferation of mobile devices, wearable sensors, and smart household appliances connected via the Internet of Things streams biometric and location data in nearly real time and at a very large scale.

Big data is a term applied to the data sets whose size or type is beyond human scale, and often beyond the ability of traditional relational databases to capture, manage, and process. Big data include information that is structured (machine readable), semistructured, or unstructured (e.g., text, video, images, audio), often with complex interrelationships. Data scientists refer to big data as having one or more distinct attributes—the so-called four Vs: volume, velocity, variety, and veracity.

Volume refers to the large scale of the data. Many of the big data sets contain a petabyte or more of information. (One petabyte could contain 200,000 DVD movies, which would take 30 years of nonstop binge watching.) *Velocity* refers to the speed at which new data are created, such as the data streaming from devices in real time. *Variety* refers to the diversity of data types—sensors, devices, video/audio, log files, transactional applications, web, and social media, for example. *Veracity* refers to the uncertainty of the data. Data have noise and artifacts, are often incomplete, often have duplicates, and can be corrupted with entry errors. Traditional manual data cleaning is a resource-intense process, often a larger task than the actual analytics. Big data exceed manual capabilities and cannot be cleaned using traditional desktop hardware and software; large-scale data cleaning tools, some that apply machine learning, are used to perform statistical audits to detect and correct anomalies.

One strategy for capitalizing on big data is using technology to aggregate data from diverse sources to create novel data sets. Geocoding, a type of geospatial analytics, uses location to link individual-level data (e.g., clinical data from EHRs and registries) and community-level data (e.g., data from the U.S. Census, healthcare claims, and nationally conducted health surveys). Nonclinical data from public records (e.g., housing, crime, human services), environmental data, and novel sources, such as Internet content from social media like Twitter and Yelp, also can be used. Such techniques can capture identity, economic, neighborhood, and behavioral factors across a variety of health outcomes. A literature review showed that this approach revealed more actionable social factors and opportunities for community interventions than analysis of single data sources.[3] Using artificial intelligence (AI) is another way to combine multimodal data. AI and geospatial analytics have been cooperatively applied to data integration with promising results for public health.[4-6]

AI and Advanced Analytics

AI is a field of computer science where machines can perform computational functions that appear intelligent. This is accomplished either by a system mimicking how humans solve problems or by a system that attains human-level performance. The foundational technologies that comprise AI in health include machine learning, computer vision, and natural language processing. While it is likely to change in the future, computer vision applications are currently being used in clinical medicine, with a few examples in public health.

Machine learning systems learn from data, rather than through explicit programming, and have achieved impressive results in healthcare. As opposed to expert systems, where humans specify the parameters of a model based on literature and informed hypotheses, deep learning can uncover hidden features (analogous to predictor variables in statistical models) and relationships within the data, often at a very abstract level, that predict outcomes. These systems are adept at handling huge numbers of variables. Deep learning has a unique strength for public health: the capability to ingest multiple, heterogeneous data types (e.g., images, text, and clinical and social data). Deep learning can extract features from each data source and combine the feature sets across data types to reveal meaningful patterns at a higher level.[7] This ability to take multimodal inputs is well suited to enhanced disease surveillance as well as analytic tasks in support of integrating biopsychosocial data into patient care.

Machine learning techniques are used for predictive analytics similarly to how a regression is used. The models can enhance population segmentation by helping to identify subgroups with common risks and health needs, allowing for precisely targeted interventions.[8] Machine learning also can improve the predictive accuracy of standard social program eligibility models, preferentially enrolling those at greatest risk.[9]

Practitioners should be cautious that biases in the underlying data are considered; otherwise, the biases will be reflected in the outcome.[10] The potential to perpetuate socially biased patterns exists because models are trained on available historical data. While there are evolving analytic techniques to assess and account for algorithmic bias,[11] people developing, testing, and using these models need to be sensitive to unexpected results and recognize bias in the data and in the experts who train the model. Practitioners must engage with the community and listen to, and include, the perspective of underrepresented and marginalized groups—those whom bias will most affect.

Natural language processing (NLP) involves teaching computers to understand human language. There are two broad uses: understanding and generating human speech (think of the automated chatbots that power call centers) and abstracting meaning from the unstructured data in written text. NLP can ingest articles, textbooks, and other unstructured information to create a library or corpus of knowledge to support human decision-making. NLP combined with search technologies also can synthesize and extract meaning from the unstructured text across numerous policy documents or summarize and uncover pertinent information buried within volumes of individual case notes. Automated methods for analyzing physician notes have been shown to enable better identification of patients' social needs than standard case management.[12]

Health Information Technology

With more complex, fragmented, and massive data sets as well as the use of more computationally intensive analytic techniques, information technology (IT) needs will change. Big data and advanced analytics need more computer infrastructure than typically is available in most clinical, community-based, and governmental organizations. Public health will face constraints on its ability to procure and maintain on-premises IT infrastructure. Therefore, cloud computing has arisen as a viable, cost-effective alternative for meeting the needs of businesses and organizations.

With cloud computing, an organization essentially rents space on remote servers. Specific functions that can be run on the cloud include storing and managing massive amounts of data, running advanced computational algorithms across dozens or hundreds of parallel computers, and running web-based applications. The cloud has several advantages over purchasing a system. Cloud computing lets organizations develop and test analytic approaches without the cost of building on-premises infrastructure. Cloud providers, such as Amazon, Microsoft, and IBM, achieve economies of scale by hosting large numbers of users on their systems.

Cloud computing offers flexibility—it can be configured to handle ad hoc computing tasks for infrequent high-intensity jobs and is adaptable to future needs. Many issues around data governance, privacy, and security can be better addressed with the tools and services on the cloud than on locally hosted systems. Hybrid clouds combine on-premises technology that may be required for security and compliance with public cloud services and can be configured to work together seamlessly.

Despite its value, technology itself can be a barrier. For individuals, lack of access to consumer technologies can bias data collection. In addition, economic and social inequalities may be worsened due to lack of technology literacy, broadband access, or mobile devices.[3] At the organizational level, adoption of newer technologies is not equitable across health departments; smaller and more rural agencies often lack access to technology and a trained workforce.

Strategic Skills for a Modern Workforce

To cope with increasing data and analytic demands and to fully take advantage of these opportunities, public health needs to develop new skills and proficiencies. At the organizational level, health departments, government agencies, and community-based organizations will need to have a working understanding of these tools. The Public Health Informatics Institute has identified three core elements of an "informatics-savvy health department": (1) an overall vision and strategy for how it uses information and IT as strategic assets, (2) a workforce skilled in using information and IT, and (3) well-designed and effectively used information systems.[13]

Leaders will need to assess opportunities as well as mitigate risks when making strategic decisions on investing in and deploying new technologies. Organizations will not be successful at navigating innovation without a deep technical expertise paired with public health expertise. Practically, this means adding a trained informatician to the leadership team who can complement more traditional IT expertise. The role of chief informatics officer has emerged as an essential position in many organizations to lead technological innovation and to ensure a strategic approach that supports public health goals.

While IT departments serve an important role for procurement and systems administration, they often do not have expertise in data science or new developments in scientific computing. System administrators might not appreciate the technical requirements to procure and integrate the specialized hardware needed to process machine learning algorithms. Decisions related to data storage and access are heavily dependent on the types of databases and analyses being used. Issues of system security, data privacy, confidentiality, interoperability, and choice of hardware all need to be informed by business requirements and how these systems will support the overall programmatic mission.

To succeed, organizations will need access to subject matter experts across an increasingly diverse array of disciplines. Public health program planners, implementers, and evaluators as well as clinicians and other subject matter experts must become sufficiently proficient in technology to interact with and use sophisticated information systems. Individuals who are cross-trained (such as clinicians with informatics training and certification) will play a valuable role.

For midcareer professionals, the type of skills needed for success depends on their current role and desired career trajectory. Most public health professionals will be required to have a general knowledge of technology, informatics, and information systems. This basic literacy entails a familiarity with the vocabulary and concepts at a level to be an effective consumer of this knowledge and to understand the strengths and limitations of technologies relevant to accomplishing their job tasks.

For those in quantitative or analytic positions, such as epidemiologists, in addition to classical statistics, data science will become increasingly necessary. Proficiency in advanced analytic techniques like machine learning will soon become essential, particularly when working with large and complex data. In the era of big data, processing and transforming raw data into useful insights requires programming skills, specifically use of automated tools to clean, standardize, and normalize data, and a deep understanding of the limitations of the source data.

Workforce needs go beyond data scientists and include a variety of roles, such as data engineer, governance, and privacy and security specialists. Public health academic programs should ensure that graduates enter the workforce with technology, programming, and informatics skills, which likely will require new training tracks in data science and public health informatics. Training programs should also target the current workforce with distance learning and certificate programs.

Meeting these modern workforce needs will not be easy and involves a two-pronged approach. In the short term, the current workforce needs to be trained. Schools, businesses, public health agencies, and nonprofits could collaborate to create the content and opportunities for executive training programs for midcareer epidemiologists, administrators, and other staff. In the long term, developing a pipeline of tech-literate public health professionals necessitates that our educational institutions respond to the field's evolution by infusing data and analytic skills into their curricula across a wide array of degree and certificate programs relevant to public health.

Conclusion

This is an extraordinary time for public health. Advances in computer sciences and technology have led to the rise in AI applications in medicine. From automating basic repetitive tasks to enhancing predictive models and decision support, AI is poised to transform healthcare and should provide the same opportunities for public health.

Policy is changing to support this transformation. There is an emerging consensus that true health improvement can only be achieved by aligning healthcare systems with public health and population-based approaches in communities. Technology will play a large role in this. Reinforcing that notion, the National Academy of Medicine recently issued recommendations calling on the federal government to develop a digital infrastructure for integrating social services with healthcare so that consumers and providers of healthcare, public health, and human services can interact.[14]

Eroding financial support for governmental agencies and over-stretched safety net providers, however, pose significant challenges to recruiting the needed expertise. Because of explosive growth in this field, there is a mismatch between supply and demand for data scientists; employers across industry sectors are having difficulty hiring for analytic roles.[15] One strategy the public sector should consider is to avoid duplicating investments already being made in the private sector and to seek out collaboration.[16] There are many examples of successful public–private collaborations, and recent developments signal a newfound willingness by business to engage with public health.[17]

AI represents a powerful set of tools that can be applied to many areas in public health, helping to solve some of our most complex problems. Of course, it's not all about the technology. Successfully leveraging these tools requires people who can manage complex data sets, who know the life cycle of data, who understand probability and statistics, who can interpret and tell a story with that data, and who understand an agency's program and policy goals. This mix of skills does not exist in one individual; thus, leaders will need to create multidisciplinary teams of public health experts, data scientists, informaticians, and IT professionals.

Big data are beyond human scale, and machine learning now exceeds human capacity in many areas. Yet knowing which tools, data types, and models are appropriate for which questions, and interpreting results with common sense, will always be human tasks. In healthcare, AI sometimes is defined as "augmented intelligence," to emphasize that achieving results from AI requires keeping humans in the loop. To do this, public health must invest in people to develop a modern, tech-savvy workforce.

References

1. Oluwakemi Ola and Kamran Sedig, "The Challenge of Big Data in Public Health: An Opportunity for Visual Analytics," *Online Journal of Public Health Informatics* 5, no. 3 (2014): 223, https://www.ncbi.nlm.nih.gov/pmc/articles/PMC3959916/.
2. Stephen J. Mooney and Vikas Pejaver, "Big Data in Public Health: Terminology, Machine Learning, and Privacy," *Annual Review of Public Health* 39 (2018): 95–112, https://pubmed.ncbi.nlm.nih.gov/29261408/.
3. Kelly Jean Thomas Craig et al., "Leveraging Data and Digital Health Technologies to Assess and Impact Social Determinants of Health (SDoH) for Public Health Improvement," *Online Journal of Public Health Informatics* 13, no. 3 (2021): E14.
4. Quynh C. Nguyen et al., "Social Media Indicators of the Food Environment and State Health Outcomes," *Public Health* 148 (2017): 120–128, https://pubmed.ncbi.nlm.nih.gov/28478354/.
5. Saba W. Masho et al., "Understanding the Role of Violence as a Social Determinant of Preterm Birth," *American Journal of Obstetrics and Gynecology* 216, no. 2 (2017): 183.e181–183.e187, https://pubmed.ncbi.nlm.nih.gov/27729255/.
6. Adam Sadilek et al., "Machine-learned Epidemiology: Real-Time Detection of Foodborne Illness at Scale," *npj Digital Medicine* 1, no. 36 (2018), https://www.researchgate.net/publication/327118890_Machine-learned_epidemiology_real-time_detection_of_foodborne_illness_at_scale.
7. Andre Esteva et al., "A Guide to Deep Learning in Healthcare," *Nature Medicine* 25, no. 1 (2019): 24–29, https://www.nature.com/articles/s41591-018-0316-z.
8. Jia Loon Chong, Ka Keat Lim, and David Bruce Matchar, "Population Segmentation Based on Healthcare Needs: A Systematic Review," *Systematic Reviews* 8, no. 202 (2019), https://systematicreviewsjournal.biomedcentral.com/articles/10.1186/s13643-019-1105-6#citeas.
9. Ian Pan et al., "Machine Learning for Social Services: A Study of Prenatal Case Management in Illinois," *American Journal of Public Health* 107, no. 6 (2017): 938–944, https://pubmed.ncbi.nlm.nih.gov/28426306/.
10. Ziad Obermeyer et al., "Dissecting Racial Bias in an Algorithm Used to Manage the Health of Populations," *Science* 366, no. 6464 (2019): 447–453, https://www.science.org/doi/abs/10.1126/science.aax2342.

11. Ravi B. Parikh, Stephanie Teeple, and Amol S. Navathe, "Addressing Bias in Artificial Intelligence in Health Care," *Journal of American Medical Association* 322, no. 25 (2019): 2377–2378, https://jamanetwork.com/journals/jama/article-abstract/2756196.

12. Amol S. Navathe et al., "Hospital Readmission and Social Risk Factors Identified from Physician Notes," *Health Services Research* 53, no. 2 (2018): 1110–1136, https://pubmed.ncbi.nlm.nih.gov/28295260/.

13. "The Informatics-savvy Health Department Self-assessment Tool," The Public Health Informatics Institute, https://phii.org/module-4/self-assessment-tools.

14. *Integrating Social Care into the Delivery of Health Care: Moving Upstream to Improve the Nation's Health* (Washington, DC: National Academies of Sciences, Engineering, and Medicine, 2019), http://nationalacademies.org/hmd/Reports/2019/integrating-social-care-into-the-delivery-of-health-care.aspx.

15. Will Markow et al., *The Quant Crunch: How the Demand for Data Science Skills Is Disrupting the Job Market* (Burning Glass Technologies, 2017), http://www.burning-glass.com/wp-content/uploads/The_Quant_Crunch.pdf.

16. Trishan Panch et al., "Artificial Intelligence: Opportunities and Risks for Public Health," *The Lancet Digital Health*, May 2019, https://www.thelancet.com/journals/landig/article/PIIS2589-7500(19)30002-0/fulltext.

17. William J. Kassler, "Turning Barriers into Benefits to Facilitate Public Health and Business Partnership" *American Journal of Public Health* 110, no. 4 (2020): 443–445, https://pubmed.ncbi.nlm.nih.gov/32159976/. 1018-0316-z.

Public Health's Essential Ingredient

Inclusive Community Engagement

MANAL J. ABOELATA AND SHEILA B. SAVANNAH

COMMUNITY ENGAGEMENT HAS LONG BEEN understood as essential to public health and community health. It is a central feature of the Public Health 3.0 initiative, introduced in 2016.[1] It also threads through the recently revised 10 Essential Public Health Services diagram,[2] in which equity is positioned as a connecting hub—a value and a core aim of all public health functions. The updated diagram and Public Health 3.0 are calls to elevate the practice of community engagement. They recognize that today's public health challenges require broad, coordinated cooperation to improve health, safety, and well-being across the population. The Public Health 3.0 framework describes public health practice that extends beyond the public health department to a diverse array of organizations: grassroots, grass-top, public, private, faith-driven, and business-driven. It implies a system with a richer, more comprehensively conceived workforce better equipped to engage with others in a journey toward systemic and structural improvements to ensure the public's health. It articulates the role of the public health department as

Manal J. Aboelata and Sheila B. Savannah, *Public Health's Essential Ingredient* In: *Building Strategic Skills for Better Health: A Primer for Public Health Professionals*. Edited by: Michael R. Fraser and Brian C. Castrucci, Oxford University Press. © de Beaumont Foundation 2024. DOI: 10.1093/oso/9780197744604.003.0020 health strategist, contributing health data, vision, and framing alongside engaged community partners and representatives from multiple sectors.

While many organizations aspire to this vision, high-quality community engagement remains an elusive practice. Issues common to public health (such as siloed funding; pressures of time-bound, project-based deliverables; challenges of getting to scale; and the demand to conduct regulatory functions and deliver safety-net services) challenge best practices in community engagement. In addition, as governmental representatives, practitioners must overcome historical mistrust and structural boundaries that separate government from community.

The COVID-19 pandemic, resounding calls for racial justice, and repeated environmental disasters all underscore the necessity for trusted relationships within and across communities to achieve better public health outcomes. Many groups grown from natural assets embedded in communities are rising to meet these challenges and are poised to be acknowledged as part of the public health ecosystem that protects and prepares their respective community.

Crises, whether a pandemic, hurricane, or other climate-related disaster, highlight the reliance on, and need for, deep, broad, and sturdy connections. But this type of community infrastructure is always critical, not just during emergencies. Inclusive, equity-centered community engagement earns and safeguards the trust of a community while also enlisting residents' knowledge, wisdom, and power to generate their own solutions. This chapter suggests that improved community engagement that works alongside smaller, organic groups that emerge from within communities lays the groundwork for more effective public health practice.

What Is Community Engagement?

Community engagement entails relationship-building, regular communication, and decision-making that involves residents, and it yields tremendous benefits. The people most likely to be impacted by the conditions that impede health, safety, and well-being are those most experienced with solutions to those problems. The

CDC's foundational Principles of Community Engagement defines this approach as: "the process of working collaboratively with and through groups of people affiliated by geographic proximity, special interest, or similar situations to address issues affecting the well-being of those people. . . . It often involves partnerships and coalitions that help mobilize resources and influence systems, change relationships among partners, and serve as catalysts for changing policies, programs, and practices."[3] The *Community Engagement Guide for Sustainable Communities* by PolicyLink and the Kirwan Institute (2012) describes "a process through which community members are empowered to own the change they want to see and involves communication, problem-solving, governance, and decision-making skills and strategies."[4] Kirwan Institute's *Principles for Equitable and Inclusive Civic Engagement* notes, "Civic engagement is more than a collection of meetings, techniques, and tools. It takes place in an environment made up of diverse people, practices, conditions, and values."[5]

> *Community participation, when it's real, is your main investment in accountability. It's your main investment in sustainability. Community participation is when, truly, you involve people in creating a mechanism for themselves to define change.*
> —America Bracho, Executive Director, Latino Health Access

From Missing Ingredient to Core Responsibility

To meet the moment of public crisis and move beyond it, we propose magnifying community engagement as a core responsibility, highlighting its value to all aspects of the public health enterprise and scaled to the level of the problems our nation confronts. Equity sits at the center of the Essential Public Health Services framework, shown in figure 19.1, Diagram A. Diagram B in this figure adds sustained community engagement as a permeable barrier to reaching the central vision of equity.

In both Diagram B and in practice, we must recognize the nature of community engagement as the critical "how" for achieving equity. By naming and magnifying community engagement as an explicit

Diagram A (below): *The Essential Public Health Services Framework*

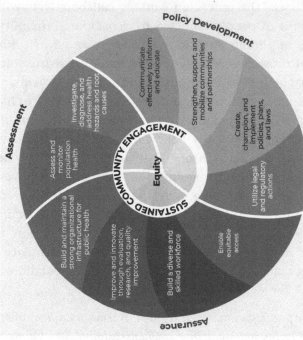

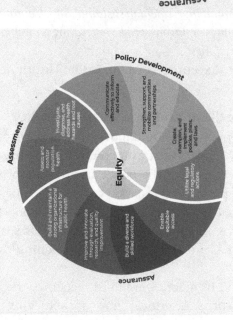

Diagram B (right): *The Essential Public Health Services Framework, magnified to identify sustained community engagement as a core responsibility and essential action for advancing equity.*

Figure 19.1. Exploring the Essential Public Health Services framework. Source: Redrawn from "CDC—10 Essential Public Health Services—CSTLTS." Centers for Disease Control and Prevention, December 1, 2022, https://www.cdc.gov/publiche althgateway/publichealthservices/essentialhealthservices.html. Public domain.

feature of the Essentials framework, we aim to elevate its importance as a key factor in all aspects of assurance, assessment, policy development, and all public health activities.

Table 19.1 lists selected public health challenges and solutions, along with questions to consider along the path to trust-based community engagement. The table is not meant as an exhaustive list; rather, it provides ideas to build on and an invitation to move toward equity-centered public health.

Toward Full Inclusion: Putting Community Engagement at the Center of Equitable Public Health Practice

Community engagement is a way of operating in service of new and better processes, systems, and, ultimately, outcomes—and not merely a strategy or tactic. At its essence, inclusive community engagement recognizes and respects the power that resides in every community. In equitable, multidirectional engagement, public health leverages its skills, functions, and resources to support the aims of community-building, social justice, and racial equity. One example that shows the impact of meaningful engagement comes from Los Angeles, as described in box 19.1.

Fully activated, public health appreciates its role in relationship to building the social justice movement and seeks to be included as an ally and a resource in reaching social justice aims. It acknowledges that trusted relationships are preexisting, and new ones are forming in communities every day. It is not satisfied with limiting public health practice to the medical or technical aspects of the field and values the social justice origins of public health. At times, public health and other governmental systems must ask to be included in those circles of trust and be willing simply to listen. An example of the impact of community-initiated engagement comes from a group of young leaders in Albuquerque, New Mexico (box 19.2).

Many groups in communities across the country are dedicated to the ongoing work of mobilizing and organizing residents and informal groups for social connection and better health. As trusted messengers,

Table 19.1. Fostering Trust to Activate Transformative Community Engagement

Barriers to Engagement . . .	Toward Solutions for Equity . . .	Important Questions to Consider	Transforming Essential Public Health Services
Lack of ongoing, authentic relationships. (Community engagement fails when it is experienced as a token gesture, box-checking, extractive, or sporadic.) Community engagement activities are often isolated or limited to public health functions, such as health education and service provision.	*Engage beyond transactional relationships.* Build sustainable relationships. Shift the focus of community engagement efforts from information-gathering to relationship-building. Use agency standing and credibility to introduce and build bridges among community partners. Sign on to policy initiatives that the community prioritizes. Recognize the value of, and invest in, community expertise on an ongoing basis. Do not ask for input unless able and prepared to consider and act on it.	• How do we support the ongoing work of grassroots and smaller organizations that are meaningful to community residents? • What are opportunities for public health to learn about and from community groups? • Who do we typically turn to when we think of our community partners? What perspectives, geographies, and racial/ethnic groups are missing? • What community workforce pathways can be built? Youth employment? Internships? Co-training with CBOs or resident groups? • How would we go about building a deeper pattern of engagement and communication?	PH 4: Strengthen, support, and mobilize communities and partnerships to improve health. PH 5: Create, champion, and implement policies, plans, and laws that impact health. PH 8: Build a diverse skilled workforce. PH 9: Improve and innovate public health functions through ongoing evaluation, research, and continuous quality improvement.

Failure to understand and address historical trauma and compounding mistrust. (Past community traumas, such as disinvestment, displacement, and violence, as well as continuing imbalances in racial and class power, create mistrust and impede connection and relationships.)

Limiting equity work to reporting disparity data rather than analyzing policies and practices that contribute to disparate health outcomes.

Yielding of public decisions to corporate influences versus ensuring public benefit of equitable health advancements.

Beyond knowing history, take actions to redress harm. Make space for healing and developing a common narrative. Take time to listen and develop a shared understanding of the community's historic dynamics and experiences. Acknowledge and allow tensions and conflict. Identify shared values and principles to foster trust. Leverage the public health voice and authority to improve community health across multiple systems. Sometimes, support rather than lead.

• What opportunities are created/supported to listen to community members without the interaction being about data collection?
• How can public institutions help validate the history of structural racism and harms inflicted by their institutions before developing solutions?
• When was the last time I, or someone from my department, attended a community forum of any kind and just listened deeply? What did I learn from that experience about how the health department might be received? Could we be a better partner?
• How do we leverage public health's influence to elevate awareness of long-standing community concerns?

PH 1: Assess and monitor population health status, factors that influence health, and community needs and assets.

PH 2: Investigate, diagnose, and address health problems and hazards affecting the population.

PH 6: Utilize legal and regulatory actions designed to improve and protect the public's health.

(continued)

Table 19.1. Continued

Barriers to Engagement . . .	Toward Solutions for Equity . . .	Important Questions to Consider	Transforming Essential Public Health Services
Discussions, processes, and places of engagement are not consistently conceived in a way that makes broad engagement possible.	*Broaden those engaged by addressing inequitable access.* Support accessibility practices and build capacity. Meet in places and times that work for community members. Ask to participate in existing gatherings. Communicate in relevant languages and take advantage of assistive technologies, from Zoom calls to translation software. Use meaningful language to engage and educate. Avoid making information and concepts unnecessarily complicated or technical. Provide skill-building opportunities to make it possible for more community members to engage.	• In thinking about my department's interactions with community residents, how often do I/we attend community forums or sit at community tables that we did not set? What can we learn from being a participant rather than an "owner" of the process? • How can trusted messengers and communication channels be resourced as part of public health message systems? • How can community messengers and communication conduits help public health use preferred media and accessible language?	**PH 3:** Communicate effectively to inform and educate people about health, factors that influence it, and how to improve it. **PH 7:** Enable equitable access.
Historically, the lead agency has controlled the decisions, budget, message, and other resources. (These imbalances inhibit meaningful participation.)	*Change power imbalances to anchor all PH services in a core of equity.* Share roles, resources, and voice. Consider different approaches, such as participatory budgeting. Invest in and be responsive to community members with leadership roles. Allow community members to shape and communicate messages.	• How well do I understand how the power that the health department wields is perceived by community residents? • What is my historical and present-day knowledge of how different actions by the health department are perceived by residents (whether coercive, neglectful, helpful, or otherwise)? • Am I able to distinguish between my own personal power and privilege and that conferred by my affiliation with the health department?	**PH 1-10:** Activate community engagement across assessment, policy development, and assurance activities to transform the public health ecosystem.

BOX 19.1. BEYOND TRANSACTIONAL RELATIONSHIPS

In 2018, a group of 20 youth leaders from the BUILD Health L.A. Initiative—a program of the National Health Foundation funded by the de Beaumont Foundation and others—conducted a comparative assessment of park conditions in multiple communities in the Los Angeles region, including their own South Central Los Angeles neighborhood. One of those youth leaders, Naomi Humphrey, described her experience: "My peers and I conducted park assessments on all 14 parks in our district using an audit tool that evaluates parks based on amenities, the condition of facilities, and accessibility." Equipped with results from their data collection, Humphrey and her peers shared their findings with community stakeholders and made recommendations to local decision makers. These youth leaders, with others, successfully advocated for equity provisions in a countywide funding measure, winning millions of dollars for communities in dire need of parks and open space. Now an alumna of the program and an undergraduate at UCLA, Humphrey continues to be an advocate for park equity, advising on community-based research and speaking publicly on issues of parks and health equity. The idea that all people affected by an issue—including young people—have a right and responsibility to participate in decision-making related to civic life is a cornerstone of democracy, and an essential ingredient in effective public health practice. Learn more in the brief *Park Equity, Life Expectancy, and Power Building* at www.preventioninstitute.org.

they can be sustaining partners in communities that bear a disproportionate burden of health inequities. The complex challenges we face today underscore the importance of acting now rather than waiting for the next crisis to adopt new ways of interfacing and partnering to ensure greater public health. Worse still would be continuing to work in isolation because engaging community is "too hard" or too time-consuming in the context of emergency response. Science tells us that we can expect more-frequent climate-induced disasters, more disease resistance, and widening inequality. It is time to strengthen community engagement as an essential feature of achieving health equity across the functions of assessment, policy development, and assurance. Inclusive, consistent engagement engenders an ecosystem

BOX 19.2. BROADENING THOSE ENGAGED

In Albuquerque, New Mexico, Together for Brothers (T4B), a small community-based organization, rapidly adapted the neighborhood-organizing efforts of their young leaders as the COVID-19 pandemic began to spread. Like many others, the group had to transition to safer alternatives that met stay-at-home orders. Within three weeks, their activities were fully virtual. Building upon existing relationships with local school and community partners, youth partners hosted ongoing social support gatherings that covered topics ranging from conducting physically distant/socially connected campaigns to bike repair, home gardening, and completing the Census. They kept young people (high schoolers and young adults) engaged in systems-change work and expanded to meet other immediate needs brought on by the pandemic—distributing food, household goods, tech support, and COVID information. The youth partners helped ensure that isolated populations within their community were reached, and they played an instrumental role as trusted messengers, information hubs, and connectors to other public agency resources. The video "How We're Staying Connected" shows how they describe this work. Find it and more about this work at www.togetherforbrothers.org.

of relationships; it enables collective efficacy and makes it possible to take on some of our most intractable challenges.

References

1. Karen DeSalvo et al., "Public Health 3.0: Time for an Upgrade," *American Journal of Public Health* 106, no. 4 (2016): 621–622, https://www.ncbi.nlm.nih.gov/pmc/articles/PMC4816012/.
2. "10 Essential Public Health Services," Centers for Disease Control and Prevention, last reviewed March 18, 2021, https://www.cdc.gov/publichealthgateway/publichealthservices/essentialhealthservices.html.
3. Centers for Disease Control and Prevention and the Agency for Toxic Substances and Disease Registry Committee on Community Engagement, *Principles of Community Engagement* (Atlanta, GA: Centers for Disease Control and Prevention, 1997).
4. Danielle Bergstrom et al., *The Sustainable Communities Initiative: The Community Engagement Guide for Sustainable Communities* (Oakland, CA: PolicyLink, 2012), https://kirwaninstitute.osu.edu/sites/default/files/2016-05/ki-civic-engagement.pdf.

5. Kip Holley, *The Principles for Equitable and Inclusive Civic Engagement: A Guide to Transformative Change* (Columbus, OH: Kirwan Institute for the Study of Race and Ethnicity at The Ohio State University, 2016), kirwaninstitute.osu.edu/wp-content/uploads/2016/05/ki-civic-engagement.pdf.

An Advocacy Primer for Public Health Practice

CAROLYN MULLEN AND LAURA HANEN

POLICY ENGAGEMENT IS A CRITICAL skill that public health practitioners can develop and utilize to achieve impactful changes in population health. Policy changes, such as indoor air quality laws, vaccination mandates, or investments in early childhood education, for example, can have a much larger impact on a community than addressing an individual's health challenges. Federal, state, and local funding for governmental public health programs—categorical disease funding for the most part—declined in the last decade, leaving little flexibility to support health department infrastructure. While it may seem beyond the scope of your job, engaging with policymakers and coalition partners is an essential role for governmental public health leaders and their staff.

While policymaking at the state and local level is a critical component of advocacy, and many of the recommendations in this chapter apply to any level of government, the focus is predominantly policy made at the federal level.

Carolyn Mullen and Laura Hanen, *An Advocacy Primer for Public Health Practice* In: *Building Strategic Skills for Better Health: A Primer for Public Health Professionals*. Edited by: Michael R. Fraser and Brian C. Castrucci, Oxford University Press. © de Beaumont Foundation 2024. DOI: 10.1093/oso/9780197744604.003.0021

Governmental public health leaders sometimes are hesitant to engage in federal policy discussions because of politics and fear of retribution from their governor/mayor/county executive or legislature/council. Moreover, many governmental public health officials receive a federally funded salary, and there is an explicit prohibition against using federal funds to influence federal, state, or local officials or legislation.[1] However, the First Amendment of the U.S. Constitution guarantees an individual's right "to petition the government for a redress of grievances." It is therefore a protected right of all Americans to lobby Congress and the administration. Before engaging in an education, advocacy, or lobbying activity, governmental public health leaders should check with their senior leadership or their governor/mayor/county executive. If the request to engage with federal policymakers is denied, governmental public health officials may take annual leave and discuss their priorities on their own time as private citizens.

Why Should Public Health Practitioners Engage in Advocacy?

While some of the most notable public health policy advancements have been achieved by patient and community advocates, there is an important role for governmental public health professionals to play in these efforts. First, public health professionals have data that are critical in making the case for policy change with federal, state, and local policymakers. Second, public health professionals are on the ground in states, cities, counties, territories, and Tribal nations and can speak to the health challenges facing their communities. Third, policymakers want to hear how laws and regulations are impacting the health of their constituents—both positively and negatively.

Governmental public health professionals need to be more transparent and accountable to both elected officials and the public about what they do every day—largely behind the scenes—to protect and promote the health, safety, and well-being of all Americans. As stewards of taxpayer dollars, public health officials should communicate to policymakers how health departments are working 24/7 on their behalf. Part of effective policy communication is helping elected officials and the public understand how states, cities, and counties use taxpayer dollars to improve public health.

One of the challenges the governmental public health community faces in advocacy endeavors is a lack of knowledge or understanding about how to advocate and why it is important, as well as the unfounded fear that advocating is the same as lobbying. Education about what governmental public health does and who it helps is related to, but distinct from, "advocacy" and "lobbying." According to the IRS, advocacy involves "promotion of an idea that is directed at changing a policy position or program at an institution." Lobbying is an attempt to influence a legislative body through communication with a member or employee of the legislative body or with a government official who participates in constructing legislation. Lobbying can include written or oral communication for or against specific legislation.

Some public health personnel are expressly prohibited from engaging in lobbying activities as part of their official duties. It is important to understand your employer's rules prior to engaging in advocacy or lobbying activities.[2] Under the Lobbying Disclosure Act,[3] providing solicited feedback on legislation or testifying before a committee at the request of elected officials or their staff is not a lobbying activity. Submitting regulatory comments is not a lobbying activity, either. A useful rule of thumb when educating federal officials is to focus on describing your programs that are supported with federal funding, both your successes and your challenges.

What Is Advocacy and How Do You Do It?

Federal advocacy is not accomplished by a single voice shouting into the void with the hope that Congress and/or the administration will listen. Rather, it is undertaken with a chorus of dedicated advocates singing loudly with one clear message. By definition, advocacy is a process by which an individual or group aims to influence decisions within political, economic, and social systems and institutions. Advocacy plays a vital role in public health. Many public health achievements can be partly attributed to advocacy for changing policy, changing laws and regulations, or increasing financial resources for implementation.

Advocacy is conducted in several ways, including, but not limited to, writing letters and meeting directly with elected officials, testifying before legislative bodies, issuing statements for the media, building partnerships with the broader advocacy community, and educating the general public so they in turn will have a desire to speak to policymakers about public health. A top priority for public health is increasing federal funding for the agencies that support public health programs at the state, local, territorial, and Tribal levels and promote policies to improve the health of the public.

Effective advocacy often is accomplished in coalition with partners—community members, healthcare providers, patient advocates, and manufacturers of diagnostics, devices, and therapeutics—working together toward a common goal. Presenting a united front across sectors can have great impact; policymakers are less likely to act if the stakeholder community is divided. This is where health departments can tap into their neutral convening role and bring diverse partners together to engage in dialogue and negotiate mutually agreeable solutions. Even in instances where health department staff are barred from lobbying, third-party validators (e.g., community and business leaders) can be essential in carrying a message to policymakers.

Advocacy is both an art and a science. There is no "one size fits all" approach, and tactics that might work in a particular advocacy campaign may not work for another. Best practices for advocacy include identifying a problem and a proposed solution, generating support and "champions" in Congress and the executive branch, and utilizing both traditional and social media to amplify the message. Advocacy also requires long-term strategy and engagement. Policy change or moving the needle on funding can take years of education and relationship-building with policymakers and coalition partners.

How Do You Put Advocacy Skills into Practice?

The following federal legislative success helps illustrate the steps in a well-designed advocacy campaign.

In October 2017, President Trump declared the opioid crisis a public health emergency. His declaration, however, did not include a request for Congress to provide additional supplementary emergency resources. National public health organizations came together to urge Congress to provide $1 billion, $500 million each year for two years, to expand population-based and community-wide public health programs. As a result of this advocacy effort, in fiscal year 2018 the Centers for Disease Control and Prevention (CDC) received a $350 million increase to support state, territorial, and local health departments in addressing the opioid crisis. Featuring a multipronged approach that included both public and behind-the-scenes efforts, the campaign combined media opportunities, a policy paper with clear descriptions of how the money would be spent, and the leveraging of relationships with legislators and the administration. Far from an easy "win," the initiative faced significant challenges. Support from the administration was not assured, since the amount of discretionary resources available was limited by budget caps, and because most federal funding for addressing substance use goes toward treatment services, advocates needed to educate legislators on the role public health plays in preventing substance use.

Before launching an advocacy campaign, governmental public health professionals need to develop a road map that encompasses seven key steps. These steps should be addressed before any conversation, meeting, or interaction with legislators, their staff, or administration officials. Policymakers' time is limited, and to become respected resources for them, advocates need to fully formulate a policy solution that includes the following key steps.

Step 1: Define the Problem

The first step is to clearly define the problem that is preventing the public from achieving optimal health. An advocacy campaign must be targeted in its approach and recognize that a multiyear effort and narrower campaign may be necessary, with achievable goalposts over time.

IN PRACTICE

For the opioid funding campaign, the problem was defined as the need for resources enabling governmental public health to address and stem the ongoing opioid crisis and the need for additional funding from CDC to scale up programming in state, local, and Tribal health departments. This "ask" was narrowly defined and focused on the role of governmental public health rather than on myriad solutions to a multifaceted and complex crisis.

Step 2: Identify Legislative/Regulatory Opportunities

Thousands of bills are introduced in Congress each year, and very few cross the finish line to be signed into law. Depending on the problem identified, a legislative or a regulatory solution can be explored. Advocates should have a clear understanding of the legislative process, whether it be bill introduction, funding and/or report language, or administrative agency regulation. Bear in mind that elections for the House of Representatives take place every two years and that champions of your effort in the House or the Senate may not be reelected or may retire. Bills from a previous congressional session die and must be reintroduced.

IN PRACTICE

The opioid funding proposal was developed as an emergency supplemental (off-budget) request outside of the annual federal funding process. Because the administration did not request supplemental funding, it became clear that an emergency supplemental bill would not progress. Advocates shifted gears to focus on the must-pass annual appropriations bills. Being nimble and looking for a variety of ways to achieve your goal increases your chance of success.

Step 3: Craft the Solution

A proposed solution to a complex problem should be researched, reasonable, well defined, and clearly articulated in a one- or two-page issue brief. Include data and graphics to convey information in a concise, attractive manner. The brief may include a menu of options to address the issue. It also may include recommendations for new statutory authority at a federal agency, formulas for how additional resources would be distributed, draft legislative language, and examples of how the policy approach would benefit and impact the health of the population.

IN PRACTICE

The opioid funding request to Congress was developed over a series of months and was informed by discussions with public health practitioners. Governmental public health advocates need to be able to justify a particular funding level and how the funding, if provided, would be directed and coordinated with other stakeholders. Those who drafted the $1 billion opioid funding request justified the amount based on recent authorizing legislation that provided $500 million each year for two years to the Substance Abuse and Mental Health Services Administration to fund state opioid crisis response grants.

Step 4: Identify Champions

To increase the likelihood of success, cultivate bill sponsors and champions from the committees with jurisdiction over public health that will ultimately act on the legislation. Committees of jurisdiction in the House of Representatives for most public health issues are the Energy and Commerce Committee, the Ways and Means Committee, and the Appropriations Subcommittee on Labor, Health and Human Services, Education, and Related Agencies (LHHS). In the Senate, the pertinent committees are the Health, Education, Labor and Pensions Committee, the Finance Committee, and the LHHS appropriations subcommittee.

IN PRACTICE

Because the opioid proposal was a funding request, advocates discussed the initiative with the appropriations committees and congressional leadership. Funding to address the opioid crisis would be determined not only by the appropriations committees, but also at the highest levels of leadership in the House and Senate in coordination with the White House.

Step 5: Build a Coalition

Most legislative successes are achieved when multiple stakeholders coordinate advocacy efforts. It is important to identify and cultivate partners in both the nonprofit and for-profit sectors and build the broadest possible coalition.

IN PRACTICE

National public health organizations worked together to amplify the need for funding of public health to address the opioid crisis through a coordinated strategy. They coordinated with stakeholders in the behavioral health and criminal justice communities, who also were seeking resources to address the crisis. Public health leaders must continue to engage with allies outside of their own sector when building coalitions.

Step 6: Take Action

Once the policy proposal is finalized and coalition partners are coordinated, the public policy campaign begins. This can include creating fact sheets and infographics, submitting sign-on letters, meeting with policymakers and their staff, and utilizing traditional and social media to amplify key messages. Typically, one organization takes the lead in developing materials and mapping out an advocacy plan. In some instances, the work is divided among organizations, with one team overseeing letters, another developing the media push, and another leading congressional strategy.

IN PRACTICE

The national public health organizations coordinated sign-on letters and scheduled visits with members on the House and Senate appropriations committees as well as with committee staff to urge adoption of the opioid funding request.

Step 7: Implement the Program

If your desired legislation does pass or funding is increased, your work is not finished. Thank your legislative champions for their important efforts, and then turn your attention to providing input on the implementation of the legislation or the distribution of the funding. This can be done formally in a letter to the agency that will implement the program or distribute the funding, or informally through dialogue with agency staff. Input may include recommendations on funding distribution methodology, program elements, and reporting and evaluation requirements. In some instances, a federal agency may be required to promulgate a rule for comment to implement a new law. Weighing in with public comment is an important way to influence the implementation process and does not fall under the federal definition of lobbying.

IN PRACTICE
With new opioid funding appropriated, advocates and the CDC discussed how the money would be distributed and the scope of allowable activities for addressing the crisis. In addition, public health organizations sent letters providing recommendations on the structure of the new funding mechanism to establish opioid prevention programs at state and local health departments.

How Is Advocacy Integral to the Future of Public Health?
Advocacy skills are essential for achieving population-level policy change and sufficient funding to support governmental public health programs. In a world of tight budgets and soaring healthcare costs, public health priorities continue to lack attention and resources. Public health practitioners are ideal messengers to policymakers in providing science- and evidence-based data to inform public health policy and funding decisions. Cultivating public- and private-sector partners to carry common messages and advocate on your behalf is crucial in tackling the public health challenges of today and tomorrow.

References
1. U.S. Department of Health and Human Services, "Federal Restriction on Lobbying for HHS Financial Assistance Recipients," 2019, https://www. hhs.gov/grants/grants/grants-policies-regulations/lobbying-restrictions. html.

2. Association of State and Territorial Health Officials, "Legal Preparedness Series," https://www.astho.org/advocacy/state-health-policy/legal-prepa redness-series/.
3. Legal Information Institute, Cornell University, "U.S. Code Chapter 26— Disclosure of Lobbying Activities," https://www.law.cornell.edu/uscode/ text/2/chapter-26.

Afterword

Leading Public Health—A Look Ahead

MARISSA J. LEVINE

Fight for the things that you care about, but do it in a way that will lead others to join you.

—Justice Ruth Bader Ginsburg

DEVELOPING THE CROSS-CUTTING STRATEGIC SKILLS detailed in this book is crucial for today's public health leaders and future leaders. Public health professionals need these skills to help shape the system and social changes needed to pursue equitable population health and well-being. Strategic skill development, though, is a process without an end—particularly in a rapidly changing world. Therefore, skill development is not just a technical pursuit. It requires the evolution of a leader's own mindset—toward a growth mindset[1] founded in resilience. Such a mindset is one that sees the opportunities presented by change and builds on strengths in a manner that inspires others to align and focus their efforts for equitable collective impact. A growth mindset alone, however, is not adequate.

Marissa J. Levine, *Afterword* In: *Building Strategic Skills for Better Health: A Primer for Public Health Professionals.*
Edited by: Michael R. Fraser and Brian C. Castrucci, Oxford University Press. © de Beaumont Foundation 2024.
DOI: 10.1093/oso/9780197744604.003.0022

Public health leaders seeking to strengthen their strategic skills must develop both their emotional intelligence[2] and a strategic mind-set[3] that builds off a foundation of strong principles (such as equity, honesty, morality, faith in humanity, and inclusivity) and values the positive (generative) relationships that are necessary to thrive individually and collectively. The leaders who first ensure the necessary mindset articulated here can then work toward defining a clear purpose for themselves. This bedrock of mindset, clear purpose, and foundational principles will position public health professionals to become the skilled strategists needed so desperately now and in the foreseeable future.

This book has highlighted the critical strategic skills needed as the third decade of the 21st century begins. This afterword highlights the book's overarching themes and outlines a vision for an aspirational future where public health leaders have developed strategic skills and use them regularly.

First, this aspirational future will happen in a world where public health work only grows in complexity—the COVID-19 pandemic being a prime example. These complex contexts will require a disciplined, yet adaptive approach to inclusive planning through engaged collaboration and effective communication. Through collaborative efforts, skilled leaders will work to develop the shared vision of the aspirational future. This vision will become the light at the end of the long, winding tunnel that allows for a sustainable collective effort despite volatility, uncertainty, complexity, and ambiguity (VUCA).

Second, skilled strategic leaders will embrace diversity and help create the conditions in which creativity and innovation are unleashed. As with the ongoing coronavirus pandemic, there will be no roadmaps for many of the issues presented to public health leaders in the foreseeable future. The leaders must probe first to sense what is happening and then, through iterative learning and adaptation of agencies and their partners, forge a collaborative path forward. Such an approach, as detailed in the Cynefin Framework,[4] is what's necessary to lead in these VUCA environments. Furthermore, public health leaders have an added responsibility to create conditions in their own agencies, through role modeling and intentional efforts to bring humanity into the workplace, that will unleash employee passion and promote joy at work. Thus, public health leaders in the aspirational future must intentionally work to create public health agencies that support and inspire the public health workforce's desire to make a difference and to do so in a way that promotes harmony and joy in the workplace.

Third, skilled leaders will work intentionally to promote aligned and focused collaboration of leaders from all sectors and at all levels of their organization and/or community. Such multisector, multiscalar, collaborative leadership will be essential to create the shared vision needed to evolve the systems that promote the emergence of equitable population health and well-being. In effect, nothing in public health happens without collaboration and partnerships, now and in the aspirational future. "Health in All Policies," for example, cannot be carried out by public health leaders and agencies alone, but represents an evolution to the Public Health 3.0 concept, where all sector leaders see their role in improving the health and well-being of the community. Skilled strategic public health leaders are the adaptive leaders of tomorrow who will ensure appropriate management but avoid being dragged too deeply into the tactical weeds, thus allowing them to spend time focusing on adaptation through strategic thinking and action. That said, through such collaborative action, our skilled, adaptive leaders, who are also fiduciary agents of public resources, could both leverage and efficiently utilize the resources available to gain maximal impact to improve the public's health.

Fourth, such leaders will also tease out the simplicity within the complexity of the issues by using the tools of systems thinking to understand the leverage points at which actions can be focused. As Meadows explains,

> There is yet one leverage point that is even higher than changing a paradigm. That is to keep oneself unattached in the arena of paradigms, to stay flexible, to realize that NO paradigm is "true," that everyone, including the one that sweetly shapes your own worldview, is a tremendously limited understanding of an immense and amazing universe that is far beyond human comprehension.[5]

Such tools enable us to both minimize the unintended consequences of our decisions/actions and better ensure we ask the right questions while avoiding so-called type 3 errors—good answers for the wrong questions. Given the significant role and complexities of communication, effective communication in an era of intentional miscommunication will require skilled leaders to connect with their communities and partners by using storytelling and other approaches that allow them to effectively relate with others as human beings first and foremost.

Fifth, these leaders, who value generative relationships, will intentionally work to create the conditions that promote such relationships, while recognizing the crucial need for diverse perspectives and inclusion to ensure the lens of health equity is always in focus.

Sixth, these same leaders will understand the role of data and evidence, their limitations as well as their interpretation and utility.

Seventh, the opportunities for implementation of technological enhancements will also be appreciated in a manner to better ensure equity.

Eighth, these skilled leaders, who are able to see, and collaborate to develop, a shared vision, will be able to articulate that vision in a manner that promotes the development of learning organizations and communities able to adapt to changing landscapes and nimbly flex funding and other business systems to meet needs.

Ninth, skilled leaders are needed who can effectively traverse the rugged political landscape in which governmental public health often finds itself enmeshed. Multisector collaboratives, or at least aligned and focused coalitions, are necessary as public health moves to become more effective in the policy arena. Policy is a critical driver of population well-being. Policy development at its heart is a relational activity. As a result, public health leaders must develop the skills to be effective actors/facilitators in that arena.

Tenth and finally, it will be important to develop authentic and adaptive leaders who can lead change while remaining focused on purpose and grounded in self and principles.

In the midst of the greatest public health challenge of our lifetime, the public health leader must be armed with the strategic skills outlined in this book:

- Effective communication
- Justice, equity, diversity, and inclusion
- Data-driven decision-making
- Resource management
- Cross-sectoral partnerships
- Systems and strategic thinking
- Community engagement
- Change management
- Policy engagement

Ideally, practitioners will approach these challenges with a "can do" attitude. This "eyes wide open" mindset will allow our skilled leaders to see the opportunities presented. Such an appreciative approach will result in working toward mobilizing others. Then, by engaging effectively and embracing our diversity and inclusivity, we will be able to chart a course toward our collective vision of a world where all people have the opportunity to thrive and maximize their well-being.

References

1. Carol S. Dweck, *Mindset: The New Psychology of Success* (New York: Penguin Random House, 2006).
2. Daniel Goleman, *Emotional Intelligence* (New York: Bantam Books, 1995).
3. Patricia Chen et al., "A Strategic Mindset: An Orientation toward Strategic Behavior during Goal Pursuit," *Proceedings of the National Academy of Sciences*, 2020, https://www.pnas.org/content/pnas/early/2020/06/09/2002529117.full.pdf.
4. David J. Snowden and Mary E. Boone, "A Leaders Framework for Decision Making," *Harvard Business Review,* 2007, https://hbr.org/2007/11/a-lead ers-framework-for-decision-making.
5. Donella Meadows, "Leverage Points: Places to Intervene in a System," The Donella Meadows Project and Academy for Systems Change, http://donellameadows.org/archives/leverage-points-places-to-intervene-in-a-system/.

Index

For the benefit of digital users, indexed terms that span two pages (e.g., 52–53) may, on occasion, appear on only one of those pages

Tables, figures, and boxes are indicated by *t*, *f*, and *b* following the page number

Healthy People 2020, 85
Heath, Chip, 76–77
Heath, Dan, 76–77
hedgehog concept, 29–30, 30*f*
Heifetz, Ronald A., 87–88, 116–17
heuristics, 131–32
HIV treatment and prevention, 26–27
homelessness, 215
human decision-making,
    understanding, 165
humility, 95
Humphrey, Naomi, 265*b*

iceberg metaphor, 43–44, 44*f*, 52
immunization, 96–97, 125–26
implementing
    evidence-based policies, 241–42
    legislation, 275–76
imposter syndrome, 66–67
inclusion
    community engagement, 261, 265*b*,
        266*b*
    diverse teams, building and
        supporting, 181–83
    moral imperative, 183–84
    in public health workforce, 178–81
influence versus authority in
    policymaking, 237–38
infodemic, 97–98, 104–5
informal versus formal data, 155–56
informatics, defined, 246*t*
informatics-savvy health department,
    251–52
information systems, 246*t*
information technology (IT),
    250–53
innovation
    examples of, 197–200
    general discussion, 190–96, 196*f*
    overview, 189–90
    in PH WINS, 33–34, 196–97
    in problem-solving, 128
insufficient data, decision-making
    with, 154
Internet of Things (IoT), 246*t*
intrinsic motivation, 141–44
intuitive brain, 165
IT (information technology), 250–53

job titles, limitations of, 172
Johnson, Steven, 199–200
Joy in Work toolkit, 144–45

justice, equity, diversity, and inclusion
    (JEDI). *See also* health equity
    leadership
    defined, 4*f*
    diverse teams, building and
        supporting, 181–83
    diversity in public health workforce,
        178–81, 178*t*
    employee engagement, increasing,
        147
    moral imperative, 183–84
    overview, 177–78
    training needs, 4*f*, 15–16
    trust in teams, 185–86
justice approach, 85

Kane County (Illinois) case study, 28, 72
Kansas City (Missouri) pre-K policy
    initiative
    background, 224
    issue, 223
    lessons learned, 225–28
    opposition to, 224–25
    overview, 223
Katzenbach, Jon, 181, 182–83
Keller, Helen, 29
Kelley, David, 193
King, Martin Luther, Jr., 219
Kirwan Institute, 258–59
knowing your ask, 219, 225
knowledge of workforce, 13–15
Kotter, John, 117
Kouzes, James M., 66
Krieger, Nancy, 85
Kuehnert, Paul, 28, 72

Ladder of Inference, 68
Laurie, Donald, 116–17
LawAtlas.org, 239
lay health workers (*promotores de salud*),
    180
leadership. *See also* change leadership;
    health equity leadership
    balancing management and, 119*f*,
        119
    collaborative, 280
    versus management, 29, 111–13, 112*t*
    mission and vision statements, 29–
        31, 32*t*
    organizational culture, creating,
        31–34
    personal, 63–64, 68–69, 69*t*